THE
EVERYTHING®
GUIDE TO
ADRENAL FATIGUE

Dear Reader,

Hello and welcome. I am thrilled that you have stumbled upon this book. Whether you picked this book up for yourself because you recently were diagnosed with adrenal fatigue, were given this book by a dear friend or relative who has experienced similar difficulties healing, or just happened upon this book and it sparked some interest, I know it has ended up in your hands for a reason.

My intention with this book is to give you the information needed to begin the journey to healing your adrenal glands. I hope the words within these pages will inspire you to reclaim your health and heal your body naturally. The world in which we live has become ridden with chronic disease and the overuse of medications to ease symptoms. The only problem is, many symptoms are not going away, and people are beginning to wonder why they aren't being treated more holistically. Now is the time for you to find the right types of healthcare practitioners who can teach you how to heal symptoms naturally. It is time to learn what it takes to heal yourself, and live a truly disease-free lifestyle.

It is my mission that each of you becomes the best caretaker of your own body, mind, and spirit. By becoming better connected with ourselves, we become better connected with each other.

You need to learn what it takes to be healthy, just as you had to learn to ride a bike or drive a car. Many people have been taught the exact opposite of what keeps them healthy. Just look at the rampant chronic disease in America. It is time you change your mindset on what heals your symptoms and, more importantly, what confers health.

By understanding how your adrenal glands and your stress response affect your health, you can positively influence not only your own health, but also that of those around you, the community you live in, and the world.

With gratitude,

Dr. Maggie Luther

Welcome to the EVERYTHING Series!

These handy, accessible books give you all you need to tackle a difficult project, gain a new hobby, comprehend a fascinating topic, prepare for an exam, or even brush up on something you learned back in school but have since forgotten.

You can choose to read an Everything® book from cover to cover or just pick out the information you want from our four useful boxes: e-questions, e-facts, e-alerts, and e-ssentials.

We give you everything you need to know on the subject, but throw in a lot of fun stuff along the way, too.

We now have more than 400 Everything® books in print, spanning such wide-ranging categories as weddings, pregnancy, cooking, music instruction, foreign language, crafts, pets, New Age, and so much more. When you're done reading them all, you can finally say you know Everything®!

QUESTION

Answers to common questions

FACT

Important snippets of information

ALERT

Urgent warnings

ESSENTIAL

Quick handy tips

PUBLISHER Karen Cooper

MANAGING EDITOR, EVERYTHING® SERIES Lisa Laing

COPY CHIEF Casey Ebert

ASSISTANT PRODUCTION EDITOR Alex Guarco

ACQUISITIONS EDITOR Hillary Thompson

ASSOCIATE DEVELOPMENT EDITOR Eileen Mullan

EVERYTHING® SERIES COVER DESIGNER Erin Alexander

THE EVERYTHING®
GUIDE TO
ADRENAL FATIGUE

Revive energy, boost immunity, and improve
concentration for a happy, stress-free life

Maggie Luther, ND

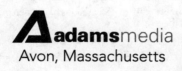
Adamsmedia
Avon, Massachusetts

An Everything® Series Book.
Everything® and everything.com® are registered trademarks of F+W Media, Inc.

Published by
Adams Media, a division of F+W Media, Inc.
57 Littlefield Street, Avon, MA 02322. U.S.A.
www.adamsmedia.com

Contains material adapted from *The Everything® Green Smoothies Book* by Britt Brandon, copyright © 2011 by F+W Media, Inc., ISBN 10: 1-4405-2564-1, ISBN 13: 978-1-4405-2564-3; *The Everything® Giant Book of Juicing* by Teresa Kennedy, copyright © 2013 by F+W Media, Inc., ISBN 10: 1-4405-5785-3, ISBN 13: 978-1-4405-5785-9; and *The Everything® Low-Glycemic Cookbook* by Carrie S. Forbes, copyright © 2014 by F+W Media, Inc., ISBN 10: 1-4405-7086-8, ISBN 13: 978-1-4405-7086-5.

ISBN 10: 1-4405-8799-X
ISBN 13: 978-1-4405-8799-3
eISBN 10: 1-4405-8800-7
eISBN 13: 978-1-4405-8800-6

Printed in the United States of America.

10   9   8   7   6   5   4   3   2   1

Library of Congress Cataloging-in-Publication Data
Luther, Maggie, author.
  The everything guide to adrenal fatigue / Maggie Luther.
    p. cm. – (Everything series)
  Includes index.
    ISBN 978-1-4405-8799-3 (paperback) – ISBN 1-4405-8799-X (paperback) – ISBN 978-1-4405-8800-6 (ebook) – ISBN 1-4405-8800-7 (ebook)
  I. Title. II. Series: Everything series.
  [DNLM: 1. Fatigue Syndrome, Chronic–etiology–Popular Works. 2. Fatigue Syndrome, Chronic–therapy–Popular Works. WB 146]
  RB150.F37
  616'.0478–dc23

2015006171

Contents

Dedication

This book is dedicated to the most amazing man I know, my dear husband Jeff, who supports me and my mission of empowering others to take care of their health in a positive way. I am also eternally grateful for our darling daughter Kaylee Simone, and for my brother and sister, parents, in-laws, last remaining grandfather, Nono, and amazing community of friends. I would not be who I am without you.

Acknowledgments

With much gratitude for my clients, I would like to thank the people in my life who make what I do all worthwhile. You entrust your healing to me, often give me the wisdom to know how to help you, and keep me learning every step of the way. While I give you the knowledge regarding how to heal, you allow me to witness healing every day. I appreciate every one of you from the bottom of my heart.

To all my teachers along the way, the ones in the classroom and those I meet on the streets, you make life worth living. I have learned countless lessons from each of you and I seek to understand how to continue to make the world the best place it can be for all sentient beings.

Lastly, to my mother, for her enduring support, always believing in me no matter how unconventional my plans sounded, and always reminding me to seek my truest path. Whether she consciously knew it or not, I have become the best version of myself because she showed me how to continue to strive for the truth.

And of course, a huge thank-you to Adams Media for making this dream a reality. I am grateful.

The Top 10 Facts about Healing Adrenal Fatigue

1. Your response to stress is what affects your health, not the amount of stress you have. Understanding this is key to truly healing adrenal fatigue.

2. Healing the adrenal glands requires an individualized treatment plan dependent on the stage of adrenal fatigue you are currently in. As you heal, your treatment adapts.

3. Inflammation and oxidative stress are the root cause of nearly all disease. Knowing how your adrenal glands contribute to these two pathologies will allow you to prevent them from negatively affecting your health once and for all.

4. The adrenal glands live in a circadian rhythm, otherwise known as the sleep-wake cycle. Balancing your circadian rhythm is crucial to healing your adrenals.

5. Nearly every system in the body is affected by poor adrenal gland health.

6. Accurate diagnosis of your adrenal glands is paramount in knowing what to do to treat and heal them. Be sure you are getting the right testing done.

7. Your diet matters when it comes to your health. To heal your adrenal glands, you will require a specific diet depending on what stage of adrenal fatigue you are in. As you heal, your diet may change.

8. Natural medicine can do wonders for accelerating the healing process and repairing broken biochemical pathways in the body.

9. Mindfulness-based practices, such as yoga, tai chi, and meditation, are necessary to transform your internalized stress response from disease-causing to health-promoting.

10. Give your body the time and right support it needs to heal. It is intelligent; when given the right diet, lifestyle, and natural therapies, your adrenals and your health can thrive.

Introduction

ADRENAL FATIGUE IS A very real concern for many people, maybe even you. When you have symptoms in your body, you have the right to understand where these symptoms are stemming from. Oftentimes people who suffer from adrenal fatigue, even the beginning stages of it, can have vague symptoms, or symptoms in various parts of the body that seem unrelated. This confusing assortment of symptoms happens because there is no system your adrenal hormones don't affect. Therefore, you may have symptoms stemming from an unhealthy hypothalamus-pituitary-adrenal (HPA) axis, and not really even know that they are related or understand that they are all coming from the same imbalance.

Because the conventional medical model does not recognize adrenal fatigue as a real condition, many people feel as though they just get sent from one specialist to another with no clear explanation of what is ailing them. This unfortunately common outcome can be very frustrating.

Adrenal fatigue is a real condition with real symptoms. You will learn all about these symptoms within this book. In addition, your adrenal fatigue may present differently than someone else's, and this is a big reason why it doesn't fit squarely into the conventional medical model. This is also why it is so important to understand how best to test for and treat the various stages, and accompanying symptoms, of adrenal fatigue. No two treatments will be exactly the same.

Most importantly, stress affects your HPA axis and is one of the main culprits causing dysfunction of the adrenal gland system. It is not stress per se that causes symptoms to arise in the body; it is your individual response to stress. When you perceive something as stressful, your body physiologically responds similarly no matter what the cause of the stress. So if you perceive standing in line at the grocery store as stressful, and you start to get tense and agitated, your body thinks you are under stress. This is not much different from how your body responds than say if you are about to get in a car accident and you really are under stress. Your body will cause the same biochemical reactions whenever you internalize something as stressful and allow those feelings to arise. The HPA axis gets activated and stays activated until you are no longer "under" stress.

The good news is that you have nearly complete control over your stress response, and that is the biggest thing you should walk away with from this book. Your ability to master how you respond to stress will be the foundation for using all the therapies within these pages, including changes to diet and lifestyle and key nutritional therapies for healing adrenal glands. Knowing what activities in your daily life contribute to a healthy adrenal system will help you produce long-term healing in your HPA axis.

Whether you know you suffer from adrenal fatigue or just have a hunch that something is wrong, this book will help you understand what stage of adrenal fatigue you have, how best to heal it, and what to do to prevent it from ever coming back.

CHAPTER 1

The Adrenal Glands

The adrenal glands are small organs on the kidneys. They are part of the endocrine system and their main responsibility is to help you respond to stress, keep blood pressure in balance, and provide the body with additional sex hormones. A healthy adrenal response is crucial to life; without one you would not survive. What happens when you perceive most of your daily activities as stressors? The body doesn't know the difference between real stress and self-induced stress. When stressors consume your everyday life, eventually the adrenal glands become exhausted. Healthy, well-functioning adrenals are crucial for every system to function normally in the body. If you suffer from chronic symptoms or a diagnosed condition, you will most likely benefit from treating your adrenal glands.

Stress, the Adrenal Glands, and the Modern-Day Crisis

Depressed adrenal function is better known as adrenal fatigue or hypoadrenia, and has become one of the major factors affecting health in the modern world. Adrenal fatigue begins when the normal stress response to acute stressful situations transitions into a heightened stress response that is maintained by routine stress. When the ongoing stress has become a daily burden, this eventually leads to a depressed adrenal response.

Reaching adrenal fatigue is most common when nothing has been done to keep the adrenal glands healthy or to restore appropriate balance when function has been compromised. You don't just wake up with adrenal fatigue one day; it is a process that takes time and develops over years of living a life where your adrenal response has become altered and dysfunctional. It is similar to driving your car around and never getting the oil changed: eventually you start burning oil, and at some point, you may even damage the engine. Your adrenal glands need regular tune-ups, preferably daily.

Adrenal Gland Disease

Adrenal gland function has been described in medical texts since the 1800s, and both overt over- and underfunction of the adrenal glands had been identified. Cushing's syndrome (hyperadrenalism) is when the adrenal glands release an excess amount of cortisol, the main hormone released when the body responds to internal and external stressors. Addison's disease, in contrast, is when the adrenal glands do not produce enough of the adrenal hormones. Addison's is referred to as chronic adrenal insufficiency.

Adrenal fatigue is not as severe as Addison's. With adrenal fatigue, there are periods of excess adrenal function that occur prior to the adrenal glands going into "fatigue," when cortisol output is excessive in response to stressors. Corticosteroids are generally not needed with adrenal fatigue, though a small group of individuals will benefit from steroids to help jump-start the adrenal gland function. In comparison, Addison's requires corticosteroid medications for survival. Both Cushing's and Addison's became well established in the medical community, as it was clear how to understand them, test for, and treat them.

Adrenal Fatigue

What isn't well understood is the middle area between Addison's and Cushing's, an area that, until recently, had been ignored and dismissed by many medical professionals. It was considered impossible for an individual to have an adrenal-related condition unless it was clear over- or underproduction of the steroid hormones. The adaptive response of the adrenals, and the ensuing disruption to biochemistry and physiology from chronic stressors, was unable to be quantified, named, and measured. Today, advanced laboratory testing and evaluation of symptoms allow practitioners and patients to evaluate for adrenal fatigue.

It is now understood that the adrenal glands will release hormones all the time when the stress response is constant. This means that the adrenal glands are being required to work continually. While the adrenal glands are meant to deal with changes in the environment of the organism, a heightened and sustained stress response makes the adrenals go into overdrive. Over time there is a constant supply of cortisol and epinephrine (adrenaline) in the blood, rather than a pulsatile amount, as is the case during a healthy adrenal response to stressors. Normally the body "pulses," or releases cortisol into the blood stream over the course of the day, with the highest amount in the morning and the lowest release at midnight.

The Importance of a Healthy Adrenal Response

Adrenal gland function and a healthy stress response are crucial to your health and well-being. Cortisol is imperative for protein, carbohydrate, and fat metabolism, as well as electrolyte balance to maintain a healthy blood pressure. It keeps your memory and focus sharp, supports nerve impulses, sustains a healthy cardiovascular system, regulates blood sugar, mediates the inflammatory response, and helps with sex hormone balance.

Adrenal fatigue does not only affect those who suffer from chronic fatigue syndrome, a more severe condition of fatigue not improved by adequate rest, or individuals who work 80 or more hours a week. Many people at different stages of their lives are beginning to see that some symptoms of their poor health are in part due to adrenal gland dysfunction. The good thing is that once you learn how to restore health to your adrenal glands and keep them healthy, you will be more likely to keep yourself in a better state of health for the rest of your life.

The Endocrine System: Your Internal Communication

The endocrine system literally means the "internal secretions." It is the name given to the hormone-secreting organs of the body, including the ovaries and testes, adrenal glands, pancreas, thymus, thyroid and parathyroid, pituitary, hypothalamus, and pineal gland. The endocrine system produces "messengers," otherwise known as hormones, which affect distant organs, tissues, and cells. *Hormone* comes from the Greek word *homon*, meaning to "excite or set into motion." This is a near-perfect explanation of what hormones do in the body; they are responsible for triggering a response from the body by causing a change to occur, by either turning a function on (excitatory) or turning a function off (inhibitory).

Once released, hormones can have a lifespan from milliseconds, as is the case with neurotransmitters, to days, more commonly seen with thyroid hormones. Hormones are primarily transported around the body through the cardiovascular system, but also travel by way of the lymphatic system, the interstitial space, and the cellular plasma. The endocrine system and specifically the adrenal glands work to make sure the organism is reactive and adaptive. *Reactive* and *adaptive* are two key words to remember in understanding adrenal gland function, stress, the stress response, and adrenal fatigue. When the body is appropriately reactive and adaptive, it means you can react to stressors and adapt accordingly, then come back into balance after a short period of time.

FACT

Stress is a normal, healthy response to a trigger. Cortisol is essential to life and has numerous biological roles in supporting a healthy body. It is only when stress and the release of cortisol are constant and chronic that symptoms of adrenal fatigue begin.

Evaluating Your Adrenal Health

When looking to evaluate how stress is playing a key role in the state of your health, you can easily ask yourself the following questions:

❑ Do you constantly feel fatigued, even after "enough" hours of sleep a night?
❑ Are you constantly in a state of worry or anxiety, or in an irritable mood, even with the ones you love?
❑ Do you have difficulty avoiding the cold and flu every year when it comes around, find yourself sick through the fall and winter season, or tend to take longer than those around you to recover?
❑ Have you been dieting, working out, eating better, but are still unable to lose weight?
❑ Do you carry around excess weight in your midsection?
❑ Do you feel tired after exercise? Do you find it hard to motivate yourself to exercise or be active?
❑ Do you suffer from a chronic condition such as hypertension, type 2 diabetes, poorly managed cholesterol, cancer, arthritis, migraines, pre-menstrual syndrome (PMS), celiac disease, Hashimoto's thyroiditis, inflammatory bowel disease (IBD), irritable bowel syndrome (IBS), chronic fatigue syndrome (CFS), allergies, insomnia, etc.?
❑ Do you go from one doctor to another being told that your lab results are normal or your symptoms must be in your head?

Stress and Your Day-to-Day Life

With regard to how you live your life, you may also find that stress is affecting your day-to-day activities, which eventually may cause symptoms. For example, ask yourself the following questions:

❑ Do you run from one thing to the next?
❑ Do you eat on the go?
❑ Do you have little time for cooking?
❑ Are you constantly thinking about what you have to do? Do you wish you did something yesterday a little differently?
❑ Are you frustrated with your life?
❑ Does your mood change, sometimes without a specific reason?

❑ Are you not in love with your job or career?
❑ Do you have a hard time prioritizing your health?

If you have checked off at least half of these in either section, then there is a high likelihood that stress, and more importantly, your stress response, is negatively affecting your health.

Modern Life Increases Adrenal Fatigue

However these questions are framed, you may arrive at the same conclusion: stress most likely consumes your everyday life, stress is a constant part of your modernized lifestyle, and the chronic heightened stress response you experience has negatively impacted your health.

The stress response in an acute situation is helpful to normalize bodily function; it helps you think clearly and act quickly. But if you live your life "on the go," it is only a matter of time before symptoms begin to appear. If you ignore your body communicating to you through symptoms, you may end up with a disease that will slowly degrade your quality of life. Symptoms that come in conjunction with adrenal fatigue can appear in multiple systems of the body or predominate one specific body system. Whether you have a symptom, have a disease, or are just on track to develop disease down the road, the one thing these questions have in common is that they tie back to the adrenal glands and the hypothalamus-pituitary-adrenal (HPA) axis. The HPA axis is part of the endocrine system, and this is how the brain communicates with the adrenal glands. Chronic stress adds to a disease state, not health, in the body. Whether you have a symptom or a disease, or have a busy life with no time to even eat a nourishing meal with your family, you are compromising the function of your adrenal system.

Symptoms and Adrenal Fatigue

Not all disease comes from stress or the effects of the stress response. Most chronic disease comes from years and years of poor health choices including dietary and lifestyle habits. However, chronic stress and your stress response are without a doubt adding to your health concerns. There is only one way to find out just how much they're contributing: by diagnosing, and then treating, the adrenal glands. You can then change your approach to your diet, lifestyle habits, and add appropriate natural therapies to suit your personalized stress response, to heal your adrenal glands, and, quite possibly, to resolve your current symptoms or disease(s).

Often people will say, "I've always been constipated," "I've always had anxiety," "I've had thin hair for twenty years," "My brain fog came when I had kids." Just because something is common or has been there forever doesn't mean it is normal, and even more so, it isn't necessarily a sign of good health. Understanding how your adrenal glands affect your health and effectively treating them will encourage improved health in the rest of your body.

Effects of Stress on the Body

Why do you need to know what stress and the ensuing release of stress hormones does to the body? So you can begin to understand that if you have chronic and heightened stress, then troubling symptoms may develop; and conversely, if you have these symptoms, there is a high likelihood that part of their underlying cause is adrenal dysfunction. Your stress response causes changes to every system in the body, and that is the key reason why it is imperative to get your adrenal health under control, to truly heal and live a symptom-free lifestyle.

Sarah's Story

Sarah came to me one day having heard about adrenal fatigue, but not knowing exactly if this was at the root of her issues. Sarah had suffered from symptoms of low blood sugar (shakiness and irritability if she went too long between meals), susceptibility to infections (routinely caught two to three colds a year), eczema, and had alternating diarrhea and constipation that had been diagnosed as irritable bowel syndrome (IBS). Sarah had read online how sometimes symptoms in multiple systems of the body could oftentimes be tied back to a weak adrenal gland system. Before coming to see me, Sarah had changed her diet, gone on the low-FODMAP diet for her IBS, and was using some natural therapies, but still wasn't seeing the results she wanted. Sarah needed help.

We assessed her adrenal gland function through a complete intake and saliva lab assessment, measuring her cortisol output at four different times over the course of the day. Adding natural therapies to help heal her digestive system, and lifestyle habits to prevent Sarah's stress from negatively impacting that area of her body, Sarah's digestive system could heal so that she did not have to continue to adhere so tightly to the low-FODMAP diet. This digestive healing also helped calm down her eczema, as skin issues often are negatively impacted by a disturbance in the health of the digestive system.

Sarah also incorporated meditation and exercise at appropriate times to help bring balance to her blood sugar. These lifestyle practices also helped Sarah better balance her stress, which further helped to heal her eczema. Healing Sarah's digestive system also greatly improved the strength of her immune system, since the majority of the immune system lives in the gut. Using ongoing targeted natural therapies for the adrenals and the immune system, Sarah is now able to stay healthy most of the year, eats a healthy whole-foods diet and has normal bowel movements, and finds her eczema rarely flares up as long as she appropriately manages her stress response.

Anatomy of the Adrenal Glands

The adrenal glands (suprarenal glands) are composed of multiple layers. The outer section is known as the cortex and the inner layer is known as the medulla. The medulla produces catecholamines: norepinephrine and epinephrine (adrenaline), which help increase awareness and alertness in the short term, as well as increase blood pressure and heart rate to be able to adapt to stressors.

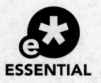

ESSENTIAL

The cortex of the adrenal gland releases hormones, which include aldosterone, cortisol, and sex hormones. The medulla, or inner adrenal, releases adrenaline. The main difference between the cortex and the medulla is that the cortex produces hormones that are necessary for life.

The cortex has three layers to it: the zona glomerulosa, zona fasciculata, and the zona reticularis. The zona glomerulosa is mainly responsible for producing mineralocorticoids, mostly aldosterone, which is the primary regulator of blood pressure. The zona fasciculata produces the glucocorticoid cortisol, which you will learn all about in this book. The zona reticularis is responsible for producing the sex steroid hormones including androgens (testosterone) and estrogens. These sex hormones are only secreted in small amounts, but as women and men age and other organs (ovaries and testes) decrease in function, the body may come to rely on the adrenals for those sex hormones.

While it is easy to say that cortisol just regulates stress and the stress response, it does a lot of other balancing activities in the body. You need to think of cortisol first as a health-promoting hormone for this reason: If you didn't have hormones, and didn't have cortisol, you wouldn't be alive. Hormones are extremely life-giving. Yet, it isn't as easy to just say, "I will remove stress from my life." Stress and your response to stressful situations is habitual, so you need to learn how to change your habits, and in order to understand how to change your habits, part of the treatment involves mindfulness practices such as meditation and yoga that help you restore balance to your body in stressful situations. Remember: it isn't the stressor but rather your response to it that is affecting your health.

Physiology and Biochemistry of the Adrenal Glands

Acute stress causes what is commonly referred to as "fight-or-flight reaction," the body's inherent mechanism of "stay and deal with the stressor or run as fast as you can to get out of there." This is often described as and best depicted in emergency situations where your life depends on you making a judgment in seconds, sometimes milliseconds—for instance, if you see a car swerve in front of you, if someone throws something in your direction, or if you are being chased by a bear. You have a strong reaction, whether that is to stay and fight or to get out of the situation as quickly as possible.

This response is predominantly mediated through epinephrine secreted by the adrenal glands. If the stress is sustained, then cortisol will be secreted. Cortisol and adrenaline release comes from a myriad of stressors on the body. They can be physical, emotional, infectious, environmental, or psychological. A release can occur when weather changes, when you get sick and spike a fever, when you are trying to avoid a car accident, or when you are sitting watching a scary movie.

All Stress Is Perceived the Same

Here is the important point: your body responds to stress exactly the same no matter what the stressor. This means that the hormones released come whether you are experiencing "good" stress or "bad" stress. The results on your physiology and biochemistry are the same. If you perceive the event as stressful, the same cascade of hormones and the effects these hormones have on various organs will still take place, until your body realizes that you are no longer under threat.

Stress Hormones

The main hormones responsible for your adrenal response include epinephrine and cortisol. The following section describes both of these hormones in detail.

Epinephrine

Epinephrine is released first when fear or anger occur. This hormone causes the following changes in the body:

- The heart rate increases so that blood can be pumped faster around the body
- The blood vessels constrict, resulting in an increase in blood pressure, secondary to an increase in heart rate with the goal of circulating the blood as quickly as possible
- Blood is primarily redirected to the muscles, away from digestive processes and urinary function, causing an increase in muscle strength and oxygenation as the muscles will be required to react promptly to move the body
- Sugar is broken down from the liver (gluconeogensis), and insulin is secreted by the pancreas to allow the sugar to enter the organs that need it: muscles, lungs, brain
- Fatty acids will be mobilized for the heart primarily, but also as a secondary source of fuel for other areas of the body

QUESTION

Is cholesterol bad?
No, cholesterol is a very important molecule for the body. Cholesterol is the base of all hormones, including cortisol, and hormones keep you alive. The body also makes cholesterol in response to inflammation, so if you experience abnormal cholesterol labs, look to reducing inflammation as a primary treatment.

Cortisol

Cortisol is released on its own and as a secondary hormone in response to a stressor, causing the following:

- As a catabolic hormone, it helps "break down" things—e.g., breaks down muscle into amino acids
- It slows down certain bodily functions—e.g., digestion, reproduction, and growth
- It alters insulin function in an attempt to prevent the released glucose, primarily from the liver through gluconeogensis, from being stored.
- It alters immune system function and exerts control over inflammatory pathways (Why do you think corticosteroids are so effective at making symptoms go away, but don't heal the underlying disease?)
- It facilitates the formation of glucose from protein

The Hypothalamic-Pituitary-Adrenal Axis

Cortisol is a steroid hormone, and specifically a glucocorticoid, produced from two cholesterol molecules. Cortisol is released when hormones from the hypothalamus and pituitary are triggered by external or internal stimuli.

When stress occurs, the amygdala, the area of the brain that contributes to emotional processing, sends a signal to the hypothalamus. The hypothalamus activates the sympathetic nervous system, which sends a signal all the way down to the adrenals to secrete epinephrine. This is the initial response to a stressor. This happens so quickly, you probably don't even know that it is happening. But when thinking about it, you may realize that your heart is beating faster, your palms are sweaty, and your mouth is dry. These are all effects of epinephrine. Once the initial response has occurred, the hypothalamus releases hormones that work through the (HPA) axis. The nervous system works in milliseconds, whereas hormones take time to get to their target organs. Having this double system set up ensures that your body can react immediately, and also that it has the ability to react in a sustained fashion, should you need it.

The hypothalamus releases corticotrophin-releasing hormone (CRH), triggering the pituitary to release adrenocorticotropic hormone (ACTH), which travels to the cortex of the adrenal glands and stimulates the release of cortisol. Cortisol will be released continually and act on target organs, until its levels are high enough, letting the hypothalamus and pituitary know to stop releasing CRH and ACTH. This is known as the negative feedback loop.

How Stress Affects Various Systems in the Body

Cortisol affects most organ systems in the body, which means that you can be sure that stress and your stress response are in part positively or negatively affecting your health. You see, health and disease exist like a seesaw: you have more of either one or the other. Sometimes the seesaw goes back and forth, and other times you may be experiencing symptoms in some areas and good health in others, a time when the seesaw remains even. However, at some point the seesaw is tipped in favor of health or disease. By evaluating and treating your adrenal glands, you can be sure to favor a tip of the seesaw in the right direction.

Cardiovascular System

Adrenaline increases the heart rate and blood pressure by increasing systolic blood pressure and lowering diastolic blood pressure. Systolic blood pressures is the top number and is reflective of the pressure of the arteries when the heart is beating. This pressure is most easily influenced by stress. Diastolic blood pressure is the bottom number of your blood pressure reading, and speaks to the amount of pressure in your arteries in between heart beats, when your heart is at rest. Cortisol has fewer short-term effects on the heart, but aids in maintaining a healthy blood pressure.

Long-term effects of stress on the cardiovascular system include sustained blood pressure elevation, edema (electrolyte imbalance), increased heart rate, thinning of the arteries, and excessive clot formation through aberrant inflammatory cytokines, all of which can result in heart attack and stroke.

Endocrine System, Specifically the Pancreas and Thyroid

Cortisol stimulates the release of blood sugar. Insulin release from the pancreas, in response to rising blood sugar, causes both utilization of glucose for energy and the storage of excess glucose for later use, including storage as fat. Long-term effects of stress on the pancreas include insulin desensitization from the ongoing release of insulin due to rising levels of blood glucose. Cortisol stimulates gluconeogensis and cortisol adverts insulin's actions by preventing glucose storage. Long-term effects of stress on the thyroid gland include both hypo- and hyperthyroid conditions. Both conditions benefit from adrenal support in addition to thyroid support for effective management and treatment, especially when looking to heal the conditions.

Reproductive System

Long-term effects of stress on the reproductive system may contribute to premenstrual syndrome and, especially in women, infertility as progesterone and cortisol follow the same pathway of production. If the body needs cortisol, progesterone will be forced to become cortisol, as it is one of cortisol's precursors. Women who experience more symptoms during menopause suffer from greater adrenal fatigue, as the adrenal glands are the chief secretors of sex hormones during this time and imbalances lead to hot flashes, fatigue, and irritability. Physical stressors may affect male fertility more, including lifestyle factors such as tight pants, bicycling, and hot tubs.

Nervous System

In the central nervous system, cortisol increases memory, alertness, and mood in the short term. Peripheral: cortisol improves muscle response through firing of neurons. Long-term effects of cortisol on the nervous system include deficits in long-term memory, mood instability, and systemic autonomic and neurological effects including numbness and tingling, nerve pain, and more.

Urinary System

Cortisol increases blood flow to the kidneys from an increase in heart rate and blood pressure on the cardiovascular system. This causes an increase in the glomerular filtration rate (GFR) of the kidneys. The long-term effect of stress on the kidneys is an increased loss of electrolytes and fluids from the body as water follows electrolytes. This can lead to an increase in blood pressure.

Gastrointestinal System

Cortisol shunts blood away from the digestive system by vasoconstriction of the blood vessels going to this system. The primary reason for this is that when you have to respond to a stressor, you are not (nor should you be) eating and digesting. Long-term effects of stress on the digestive system are indigestion, gas, bloating, reflux, malabsorption, dysbiosis (also known as dysbacteriosis, a microbial imbalance), IBS, and IBD.

Musculoskeletal System

Cortisol will increase amino acid breakdown from the muscles in order to convert them into blood sugar. This involves the transformation of amino acids into glycogen by the liver and the breakdown of glycogen into glucose for the muscles, including the brain and heart. This will permit the muscles to react in milliseconds if necessary.

Long-term effects of stress on the musculoskeletal system can increase arthritis, muscle cramping, and excess blood sugar stores in the muscles. Cortisol will trigger release of triglycerides from storage and deposit them into the visceral waist fat. Chronic effects of stress on the bones include a reduction in calcium absorption in the intestine and an increase in calcium excretion by the kidneys, both of which negatively affect the protein matrix of the bone, leading to weaker bones.

Immune System

Cortisol helps to modify the immune response by increasing appropriate immune responses in reaction to a stressor, such as increasing anti-inflammatory pathways. However, long-term effects of stress on the immune system include overstimulation of the anti-inflammatory pathways, leading to eventual reduction and a malfunction of the immune response, resulting in ineffective immune system reactions when the time is necessary. Those with a lowered adrenal response tend to get sick more often, stay sick longer than peers, experience allergies and/or asthma, and may experience autoimmune conditions.

History of the Term "Stress"

A man by the name of Hans Selye coined the term "stress" in the 1920s. Selye, an organic chemist, had observed that people with different diseases exhibited similar symptoms, such as loss of appetite or low energy, causing them to look and feel sick. At the time, the medical paradigm believed that nearly all illnesses were caused by pathogens, with tuberculosis, syphilis, and other communicable diseases being on the rise.

In his lab, Selye had noticed that animals would respond with similar physical and pathological symptoms, including stomach ulcers, changes in immune cell response (shrinkage of lymphoid tissue), and enlargement of the adrenal glands, when exposed to stimuli such as bright lights, loud noises, and drastic changes in temperature. Selye demonstrated that when these stressors were continually applied to the animals, resulting diseases, which mimicked chronic symptoms in humans, began to form, including heart disease, stroke, kidney disease, and rheumatoid arthritis.

FACT

Hans Selye was the first to define stress as "the non-specific response of the body to any demand for change." This has become the most common way to define stress, although some feel that the intricacies of the stress response are lost in such a simple definition.

Selye went on to describe this phenomenon as General Adaptation Syndrome (GAS), a response from demands put on the body over time. The syndrome explained how stress causes a host of autonomic changes within the body, and how these changes lead to various disease states, either directly or indirectly from various systems malfunctioning. These processes, Selye explained, involved hormones and the endocrine system at large, but specifically were directed by the adrenal glands. Selye's work went on to explore and extrapolate how the syndrome was at the center of the same diseases he had demonstrated in laboratory animals. In humans, these stressors could lead to ulcers, high blood pressure, allergies, arthritis, nervous system aberrations, and kidney disease.

Selye helped the medical community and greater public understand the difference between stress and stressor, as the former has positive effects on health, whereas the latter term could be used to distinguish something that could cause ill effects on the organism. Good stress later came to be defined as eustress. For instance, a roller coaster ride, winning the lottery, giving a lecture or presentation, or going on a vacation all affect physiological changes in conjunction with the stress response that are normal and healthy. It is only with a stressor such as living a hurried life, always feeling late, or dreading a conversation with a boss or loved one that the stress becomes problematic.

How Two Little Organs Do So Much

The adrenal glands are two relatively small organs, one sitting on top of each kidney. Each is no bigger than a walnut, and weighs on average 2 grams. Don't be fooled by the size, though, because the function the adrenal glands have on normal homeostasis, or the body's ability to respond and adapt to stressors in the environment, is quite impressive. They are right up there among the most important organs you have. While organs such as the heart and brain are essential to life, the adrenal glands serve as the conductor keeping the whole orchestra of body systems coordinated and smoothly playing the song together.

So if you feel tired, worn out, or just can't get enough energy to carry you through the day no matter what you do, then you are in for a treat. Understanding how you can restore health to your adrenal glands and help your body heal symptoms, stop diseases from progressing, and prevent chronic disease is one of the greatest gifts you can give yourself. This book will help you figure out how to do that.

Understanding how to appropriately diagnose adrenal fatigue, knowing what you need to do as an individual, and using the tools including your everyday habits, diet, and lifestyle will greatly improve your quality of life.

Treating the adrenal glands and the stress response is becoming a more common first step in the restoration of health. Given the right combination of natural health, dietary adaptations, and transformations in lifestyle habits, including (most importantly) mindfulness practices, you too can achieve restored adrenal gland function and gain back energy, vitality, and youth, and feel great again.

Please note that the words "stress" and "stressor" will be used interchangeably, with the intention of both representing a stressor placed on the body: running a marathon, avoiding a car accident, giving a presentation, running from one event to another, etc. All these events place a stress on the body, and it is your response to the stressor that matters most when healing your adrenal glands.

CHAPTER 2

Your Response to Stress Matters

Stress is defined as a physiological response to an external stimulus. A stress placed on the body triggers a whole host of reactions, beginning in the brain, ending in the adrenal glands, and resulting in systemic physiologic changes. Hormones, neurotransmitters, and the nervous system are all "on" when the stress response is activated. Meeting one's basic needs can be stressful for many: Where is your next meal going to come from? How are you going to pay the rent this month? Yet, you don't have to be just thinking about your basic needs being met to experience the ramifications of your heightened stress response. Anytime you go into "stress mode," you will experience symptoms of a dysfunctional adrenal response. Your adrenal health depends on how long you let the symptoms go before you create some positive lifestyle changes to help reduce the mental trigger of stress mode.

Stress: For All It's Worth

Stress is a normal part of everyday life, but your response to stress could be having a detrimental effect on your health. Maybe not today, maybe not tomorrow, but inevitably your stress response is causing you more harm than good. Stress is hugely subjective, as there are vast differences between individuals as to what defines a stressor. Even within the same individual at different times or situations in life, a stress may be perceived differently. For instance, you may perceive being stopped at a red light as stressful, while another person stopped at the same red light is totally enjoying the song on the radio. Likewise, you may feel very different if you were to lose your house at the young age of 25 versus age 65.

Stress has become an everyday word in twenty-first-century life. Not only are you affected by stress on a daily basis with all the various commitments you have, but you have placed yourself "under stress" as a way to deal with just getting by in life, living day to day. For instance, how common are these thoughts in your head:

❑ "I feel stressed."
❑ "I am constantly running from one thing to the next—this is stressful."
❑ "How are we going to pay the bills this month? I am just so stressed out over money!"
❑ "I don't have time to cook dinner at a reasonable hour. I have to stay late—I am under too much stress at work."

Your Mental Response to Stress

Your thoughts influence your biochemical and physiological processes. You are stuck in the cycle of having a stressful thought and actually feeling the hormonal trigger. Instead of having the thought and letting the thought go, your body picks it up as its cue to trigger the hypothalamus to say, "Hey pituitary, tell the adrenal glands to respond." After all, you're under stress, right? The body is just doing what it knows best to do . . . respond!

You're really not under an actual life-threatening stress; you're under a psychologically induced stress, a mental stress. This is also true of an emotional stress. Picture watching a scary movie: What does your body do? Your heart beats faster, you get anxious, you react to any noise or movement.

Every time you respond to something as a stressful event, you are conducting an experiment on your physical body. And the problem with that is, too many experiments will eventually wreak havoc on you physically. This is why it is your response to stress that matters so much! The good thing about this scenario, though, is that you don't necessarily have control over stress, but you *do* have control over your stress response.

Why You Should Care

There is a misconception that stress is something benign, or that it is somehow out of your control. You know that stress isn't good for your health, but you're not really sure what that means. Instead of looking at stress as something that is happening to you, begin to look at your stress response as something that is happening within you.

Every time you get stressed out, you are causing the same physiological response in your body as you would if your life were really in danger. Your mind doesn't know the difference, and therefore, your stress response must be healed in order for you to feel well again. This is not simply about taking something to make your adrenal glands function better; that can help, but ultimately you will need to practice changing your mindset. You must learn how to effectively alter your perception to stress and stop causing your body to be in continual fight-or-flight mode. You must learn how to calm down the adrenal and nervous systems so that your body is balanced between acute stressors and healing. You will learn how to do this by flipping your disease-promoting habits into health-promoting habits.

ESSENTIAL

Remember that your response to stress over time can cause a whole range of symptoms and contribute to chronic conditions. Therefore, it is highly likely that if you struggle with anything health-related, some part of it has to do with your response to stress.

Your Response to Stress Creates Disease

What is now observed, recognized, and substantiated, in conjunction with what Hans Selye attempted to define about stress, is that there is stress and there is the stress response. While these two pieces are intricately connected, you have control over one and not the other.

Given that stress itself can be quite healthy for survival and allows you to complete a task or finish a project, current scientific findings demonstrate that it is not necessarily stress itself that is the enemy, but rather your response to stress (or a stressor) that is much more important to your state of health. Better put, disease is more likely to be a ramification of stress based on your response to stress, not simply stress.

The good news is that in the long run, you have the ability to learn what it takes to adapt your response to stress, and that is a much "simpler" task than to try to make all stress go away. That just isn't going to happen, unless you wake up on some remote island in paradise. But then you would probably have to worry about where your next meal is going to come from.

Physical, mental, and emotional symptoms caused by an ongoing elevated response to stress include some of the following:

- Anxiety, confusion, irritability, hair-trigger temper, frequent agitation
- Difficulty quieting your mind, inability to relax, constant worrying thoughts
- Chest pain and/or heart palpitations
- Muscle aches or pains, headaches
- Upset stomach leading to heartburn, constipation, diarrhea, loss of appetite, change in appetite, clenched jaw or grinding of teeth
- Frequent colds or infections
- Loss of sex drive, apathy, depression
- Inability to focus, poor judgment, lack of follow-through on commitments
- Increased need for stimulants and/or relaxants
- Nervousness, shakiness, changes in body temperature, fidgeting, pacing, nail biting
- Seeing only negative outcomes in life, feelings of loneliness, isolation, distance from others

Can you believe these can all be caused by stress? This is why it is important for you to *want* to understand how stress is not some arbitrary thing that happens outside of your control. The way you feel today is a direct reflection of everything you have done up to this day, and some part of your stress response is to blame.

Your Stress Response over Your Life

What stressors have you had over the course of your life? The death of a loved one, not getting promoted at your job to a position you deserve, an automobile accident, raising a family, juggling a career and climbing the corporate ladder, getting ill, etc. The list really could go on. And after each event, the goal would have been that you *effectively* processed the physical, emotional, and mental trauma from the event and you took time for yourself to heal. The problem is, no one ever really does this. Instead, one after another, the physical, mental, and emotional stressors take their toll on your body and you are never able to fully recover after each one. Remind yourself: you desperately need down time.

Your Stress Response Gone Wrong

Think about all the things you consider stressors in your life. They could be ones you create, such as getting stressed when you wait in line at the grocery store, or ones that you feel are imposed on you, such as deadlines at work. How common is it for you to be stressed: daily, hourly, most of the day? Take a look at the following list of stressors. Do you fall prey to feeling "stressed out" in the following scenarios regularly?

❏ You are late to the big meeting with your boss and the CEO of the company; you are up for a promotion and you suspect this meeting is part of the evaluation process to see if you are ready.

❏ There are five people ahead of you in line at the grocery store and there are only two people working the cash registers, both lines equally as long.

❏ Your to-do list is about a mile long, it is 4 P.M. and you only have 30 minutes until the kids are home, you have to make dinner, and there is a school meet and greet this evening. You just realized you are out of two ingredients that you were going to use to make dinner.

You actually have the choice to live with a revved-up stress response or, beginning today, to get your stress response under control.

The Road to Adrenal Fatigue

By now, you know that when you experience a stressful event, you acutely respond to the stress by releasing a whole host of hormones and neurotransmitters, causing a slew of biochemical reactions throughout the body. Over time, your adrenal response gets elevated as you ask it to respond over and over again; your body responds for years in a heightened state, pumping out cortisol, and you are in a "hyper" adrenal state. Eventually your adrenal response "drops off," and you are left with adrenal fatigue, hypoadrenia.

Your body has responded to perceived stress for a very, very long time; you are too exhausted to respond anymore, be it from lack of nutrients, inability to cope, inappropriate lifestyle choices, poor dietary choices, or mental and/or emotional trauma. In fact, it is extremely common for the "breaking point" to come in the form of an emotional grief, sending you right into adrenal fatigue.

A study written up in 2014 in the *Journal of Psychosomatic Research* concluded that individuals who experienced burnout symptoms had a lowered salivary cortisol output, supporting the fact that when the stress response is ongoing and the individual experiences symptoms, eventual cortisol depletion will occur. Symptoms don't lie!

Stop with the Autopilot Life

Some people wake up, grab a cup of something caffeinated, start rushing through the day, bouncing from one stressful situation to the next, get home to dinner, use some sort of sleep aid and go to bed, only to wake up tomorrow to do it all over again.

One major problem with such an overloaded routine is when one of those big stressors comes along, you don't take the time you need to fully recuperate. You are left with a little bit less reserve in your adrenal gland tank each time. Eventually, the tank is empty and you are running around still in exaggerated stress-response mode, but your adrenals have nothing left to give. Equate this to a dying battery in your car—you try to start it, but the starter just revs and doesn't turn over. There is no more electricity left for you to turn your adrenals on and this is a problem.

Change Your Mind, Change Your Life

You respond in a specific manner to every event you perceive as stressful in your life. Your body physiologically does not recognize whether you are in true danger (e.g., running from a saber-toothed tiger) or if you are just making up the danger (e.g., stuck in a traffic jam). So every time you go into "stress mode" you are causing your body to respond with a flood of hormones including cortisol and adrenaline. Then your body must respond to these hormones and do the following: break down blood sugar for muscles to use via the liver, break down amino acids from muscles to convert to glucose and store as glycogen in the liver, shunt blood away from "unnecessary systems" such as digestion and reproduction, and pump blood to critical organs including the brain, heart, and skeletal muscles to enable quick reactions. And the cycle continues while you are under the stress you have imposed on yourself. In order to change how stress negatively affects your health, you have to open your mind to the possibility that you are actually *in control* of how you *respond* to stress. So for instance, next time you are late to a meeting, try doing some deep breathing and calm your mind down on your way there. You are already late—you can't change that. This won't be easy, but each time you recognize that you consciously can respond differently to how you feel under stress, the less stress will harm you.

Give Your Body What It Needs

Your body can only heal when you are truly resting. Why do you think sleep is so important? Because your body is repairing itself overnight. Your endocrine system is hard at work releasing growth hormone, thyroid hormone, and adrenal hormone so that your body can prepare itself for the day to come. Remember, your body is innately intelligent; you just need to give it a chance to fully recover from each day. Now, you can't sleep all day. However, you do need to restore health to your body and you need sleep and relaxation to do that.

Take Sally, for example. Sally was a 51-year-old female who was exhausted, anxious, and irritable. She had been sleeping poorly for the past decade and was heading through menopause miserably. Hot flashes, anxiety, and irritability were rampant. She was also carrying around an extra 10 pounds of weight in her waist, one of the major signs that poor adrenal function is affecting your health, and had mild hypertension. Sally was desperate to help herself feel better and was tired of yo-yo dieting, not experiencing lasting change.

Focusing on hormones, including the adrenals, by helping the liver process the hormones using liver supportive herbs, and a natural fiber supplement, Sally was sleeping better in just 2 weeks. In fact, she had been sleeping better than she had in the last 10 years, and experiencing less irritability. She had also lost 5 pounds. All of this was accomplished with dietary and lifestyle changes to support healthy adrenal glands and adrenal response, as well as specific nutrients and herbs for her specific nutrient deficiencies. Sally went on to lose all the weight she had wanted to, continued to experience full nights' sleep, lowered her blood pressure, and came off of her blood pressure medication all because she focused on healing her adrenals and her hormones, as well as supporting weakened systems.

The Good News

Researchers at the University of Wisconsin–Madison asked almost 29,000 people to rate their level of stress over the past year as well as report how much they believed this stress influenced their health—a little, a moderate amount, or a lot. Over the next eight years, public death records were used to record the passing of any subjects.

People who reported having high levels of stress and who believed stress had a large impact on their health had a whopping 43 percent increased risk of premature death. On the other hand, those who experienced a lot of stress but did not perceive its effects as negative were among the least likely to die prematurely compared to all other participants in the study. Individuals who perceived that stress affected their health a lot had an increased risk of premature death.

This research really shows you how your response to stress, and not the stress itself, will harm your health negatively. When you create a stressful situation in your mind, you create the cascade of stress hormones being released.

What Is the Solution?

The best way to combat stress is to learn how to challenge your response to stress. Instead of just getting flustered, hot and bothered, annoyed, irritated, withdrawn—whatever your "go-to" place is when you are under stress—stop, take a deep breath, and begin to ask yourself what you can change about how you are responding. Chances are, you can change a lot. And what this translates into is a foolproof way to get your stress response under control and reclaim your adrenal health.

Let's look at Fred as another example. Fred is a 46-year-old male who has suffered from depression, anxiety, IBS, and difficulty with focus nearly his entire adult life. Fred had a management position in his company and his primary responsibility was event planning. Talk about stressful.

Fred had previously turned to both conventional and holistic/complementary healing practices over the years to help him with his symptoms. The problem was, Fred had incurred so many stressors over the years that were not appropriately healed that his symptoms were only being managed. Anytime he tried a new therapy, either pharmaceutical or natural, the treatment would work for some time but then slowly stop being effective. Fred was fed up.

Fred's adrenal response was in the burnout/hypoadrenia state, he was barely making it through the day because of the level of fatigue he experienced. A simple salivary cortisol test showed low cortisol output throughout the day, with a spike before bedtime, which of course was contributing to poor sleep quality, a symptom Fred was just "dealing with." Fred needed specific help with his ability to manage the stress he would continue to face in his management position.

Along with specific dietary and lifestyle recommendations, natural supplements specific to healing the digestive system and the adrenal response, stress management techniques, and continual support, Fred was able to become better aware of when his stress response was negatively affecting his health. Fred's IBS healed, his anxiety quieted down, and his depression and his focus both improved, allowing him to come off his medications. He was better able to rely on natural therapies to help weather the more stressful times in his job. Focusing on healing, Fred was able to restore health to his adrenals, mitochondria (the energy producers of all cells in the body) and brain function. Fred felt like a new man, not only because his symptoms were healing, but also because he had become better educated at how to deal with his stress response so these symptoms would stay healed.

What You Can Do

The symptoms of adrenal fatigue are many, as you have seen, and your body's ability to heal is dependent on two conditions: (1) you give yourself the right support to heal the adrenals and other systems experiencing symptoms with specific natural therapies, diet and lifestyle modifications, stress management techniques, etc. and (2) you learn what you have to do in your daily life to transform your response to stress so that it no longer harms you.

How to Change Your Relationship with Stress

In order to take back control of how your stress response is affecting your health, first you need to figure out what routines in your daily life cause you to be "stressed." Could it be doing chores around the house, talking to your boss or partner, interacting with your children, worrying about finances, standing in a long line at the grocery story, waiting at a red light, juggling work and household demands—or all of the above?

Start Now

The easiest way to start managing your stress is to identify the things you do day in and day out that make you worried, anxious, nervous, or irritable. These are the things that you can tackle first. What you will do is begin to identify when you are heading into stressed mode. So let's start with an example. Say you are stressed every time you drive home from work. It's been a long day, you have a 45-minute commute that is filled with traffic, and you have to deal with the family and make dinner when you get home. You have to do this every weekday; there is no way around it. Well, the most effective way to immediately stop this from negatively affecting your health is to recognize that you, you, and only you, have the power and ability to challenge how you react to this situation.

Next time you are driving home, try this one on: First identify that you are stressed because you are sitting in traffic, you can't get home any faster, and you have to cook a meal once you do arrive home. Accept that this is the truth. After all, it is! Maybe even wallow in the fact that this is the truth. It is okay to be sad and disappointed that when you get home your time is not your own. Then, take three deep breaths and continue to accept this reality. You cannot change the reality of where you are, but you can change your response to it. Stop thinking about everything you still have to do and enjoy the drive home. Here are a few ideas:

- Find an audio book series you can listen to. Hey, it can even be one on stress!
- Take a different route home: maybe you realize that what you dislike most about your commute is sitting in traffic on the highway. Maybe you could find a back road to get home if you can. You may really enjoy the scenery.
- If you don't like driving, find someone to commute with. You may be surprised to find that someone at your workplace lives within 5–10 minutes of you; you could end up alternating driving duties with a coworker.

Your Chance for Change

Stress in and of itself is not a bad thing. Stress helps you cope with life by making you think more clearly, focus better, respond more quickly, and react to a present situation. Acutely! Yes, you need the stress response to live. What you don't need is an aberrant stress response to nearly everything in life.

The goal is to learn how to live with stress and adapt your response to stress so that you are in control of it, rather than it being in control of you. This can be done. It takes consistent work and mindfulness in reframing what you believe to be stressful. You will find that a big part of changing the way stress is affecting your life is coming to terms with how you live and perceive the world. First, just begin to get comfortable with the fact that you have the power to change your stress response.

CHAPTER 3

How Your Stress Is Affecting Your Health

When the body is constantly under stress, you engage your stress response over and over again. That would be okay if you lived in a world where you could allow your body the time it needed to recover from each stressor, but most people barely have enough time to relax at all. It is your response to stress that influences your health, not necessarily the stress itself, so you can learn to correct your stress response and support your health.

Your Body's Response to Chronic Stress

At this point you may be thinking, "So what, I have stress, I doubt it affects my health that negatively." Well, you may have a different answer after reading this chapter. Stress causes different hormones and neurotransmitters to continually be released around the body. The body responds and responds, as quickly as it can, to all these chemical messengers. Eventually, though, not only do conditions such as oxidative stress and inflammation increase, but your cells start to become desensitized to communication.

The best example of this is with type 2 diabetes (DM2). Part of the pathology with DM2 is that over time, your pancreas has been "asked" to release insulin continually, because of a combination of unhealthy dietary and lifestyle choices, poorly managed stress, and genetic factors. The cells in the body are exposed to the insulin too much. Suddenly, or more likely over years of exposure, the insulin receptors on the cells begin to not be able to utilize the insulin anymore. So, what does your pancreas get told to do by the brain? Make and release more insulin.

One of the main early pathologies of DM2 is elevated insulin. Stress negatively affects DM2, as cortisol is designed to increase blood glucose. *Glucocorticoid* means "glucose" corticoid, so one of the main roles of cortisol is to increase blood sugar. This makes sense if you remember that your muscles, brain, and heart will need glucose to react quickly to whatever stressor is causing the cortisol release.

Similar to insulin desensitization, cortisol can also follow the same path, where the cortisol receptors stop responding to the increased load of cortisol in the body. This often happens on the way to adrenal fatigue, during stage 2, where overproduction of cortisol is common. When you run a salivary lab test at this stage, your cortisol will be elevated during certain times throughout the day, and may also be low at abnormal times (e.g., in the morning).

Eventually, if things continue in your current state of adrenal fatigue, the majority of the salivary measurements over the course of the day (there are four) will become depressed. This is exactly what happens with the pancreas. Once it puts out excess insulin, eventually it stops putting out enough insulin at all, and many advanced DM2 patients will need insulin injections.

Oxidative Stress and Inflammation

Oxidative stress is a term used to describe an imbalance in the body's generation of free radicals and reactive oxygen species, with an appropriate balance of antioxidant defense systems. Free radicals are generated both by the body and from exposure to things from outside the body. When new cells are made or when the cells make energy by way of the mitochondria, where oxygen is converted to ATP, the main form of energy in the body, free radicals are created. When you are exposed to heavy metals, toxins, or noxious chemicals and gases, you are exposed to free radicals. Inflammation, on the other hand, is your body's ability to create an inflammatory response to something, be it a pathogen, irritant, or something the body produced (e.g., a cell). Oxidative stress is implicated in nearly all disease, and so is inflammation.

Oxidative stress and inflammation may be mutually exclusive in how they develop in the body. One is involved in the generation of free radicals and the other is a biological response to a stimuli. Both are necessary to healthy living, and yet both can be completely out of control. You will want to know what this means for you and how something that is normal can also have the potential to become so destructive.

Adrenal Health, Oxidative Stress, and Inflammation

When appropriately treating the adrenal glands and adjusting how they ultimately function, it is important to consider an imbalance in the oxidative stress and inflammatory pathways. Much of the time this is not considered or addressed when treating the adrenal glands, and then the adrenals don't get everything they need to become fully restored and healthy. Oxidative stress and inflammation is best treated by way of the diet and lifestyle, by adding in more fresh fruits and vegetables, exercising regularly, getting fresh air daily, and much more. When you just focus the treatment on adrenal glands, the powerful benefits of reducing inflammation and oxidative stress through your daily habits, diet, and lifestyle, you don't get as much recovery in your health.

The adrenal glands are *extremely* busy organs. They produce cortisol, aldosterone, and sex hormones, essentially all the steroid hormones. It takes a lot of oxygen to keep the mitochondria of these cells producing the energy they need to keep going. Mitochondria are the energy producers of the cells and are necessary to keeping the cell alive. In the process of using oxygen to create energy, mitochondria will create free radicals

Steroidogenesis, the creation of steroid hormones, is very energy intensive, and thus your adrenals themselves are at risk for damage from an imbalance in the oxidative-antioxidant system in the body. The creation of new steroid hormones causes oxidative stress to occur and inflammatory pathways are elicited, increasing the amount of inflammation present. To make matters worse, everywhere there is inflammation, your body needs to release more cortisol to help calm down the inflammatory response.

ALERT

Inflammation causes oxidative stress because inflammatory cells need oxygen to make energy to survive. When your body is chronically inflamed from a poor diet, lack of exercise, no hydration, and poor lifestyle habits including nonrestful sleep, you produce more inflammatory cells and more reactive oxygen species. If you don't get control of your inflammation by eating a healthy diet, exercising regularly, breathing fresh air, drinking clean water, calming your mind, and so on, you will only be producing more free radicals your body has to deal with.

If your adrenal glands are overwhelmed with oxidative stress, causing free radical generation and increasing inflammation, then your adrenal glands are not going to function ideally. You will be asking more and more of your exhausted adrenal glands, which are not healthy themselves. How can a weakened organ support the whole body? Simply put, it can't. And eventually you will notice how your health is affected. Therefore, improving your body's oxidative stress balance and inflammatory response are also key to restoring adrenal health.

Oxygen: The Good and the Bad

Oxygen (O_2) is both a necessary good and an evil. Human beings absolutely need it to live, every single moment of their lives. You use oxygen in the mitochondria of your cells to make adenosine triphosphate (ATP), the energy that runs the cell. You also use oxygen to support other metabolic pathways, including cellular proliferation and differentiation, apoptosis (cell death), immune regulation, detoxification, and cellular adaptation to stress.

Oxygen creates free radicals; it is a normal part of biological living in all aerobic ("with oxygen") pathways. Chemically speaking, any molecule that contains an unpaired electron will want to find another electron to become "stable." Oxygen contains two unpaired electrons in its orbit. And the reason those two don't pair up is because each is in its own orbit. Therefore, both will look for electrons to become stable. In the body, O_2 takes part in numerous electron-accepting and electron-donating reactions.

How Oxygen Creates Free Radicals

One of the reactions in the body where oxygen accepts electrons and produces free radicals is in becoming water. The first thing oxygen becomes when it accepts a free electron is superoxide radical (O_2-). This molecule is a very destructive free radical produced by your body, and is so unstable because the oxygen still has one unpaired electron. It will be looking for one to take from somewhere else, and it isn't selective.

The body is pretty smart and is able to donate an electron and two hydrogen atoms as needed from your antioxidant system, causing the superoxide radical to become the non-radical hydrogen peroxide (H_2O_2). While this is not a free radical per se, it has the potential to generate free radicals, as you will see shortly. But at least the body has neutralized the more reactive and destructive O_2-.

However, hydrogen peroxide can interact with another electron and a single hydrogen atom to form water (H_2O) and a hydroxyl radical (OH-). This is good because the body has produced water, but now it has to deal with a second free radical similar to superoxide radical in reactivity and destruction of anything it interacts with. With the addition of a fourth electron and one more hydrogen atom, the hydroxyl radical will form water.

Reactive oxygen species (ROS) are generated in healthy pathways in the body, including when oxygen becomes water. ROS are free radicals that can get out of control and cause inflammation if not appropriately balanced by the antioxidant systems in the body. In a healthy person, roughly 3–5 percent of the oxygen you consume is destined to form free radicals.

Other Forms of Oxidative Stress

On top of ROS, there are also RNOS, which stands for reactive nitrogen oxygen species formed from nitric oxide (NO). Nitrogen is nearly as prevalent as oxygen in your body, and RNOS, including radical nitrogen dioxide and the non-radical peroxynitrite, are active in our blood vessels, working to vasodilate (widen) the arteries and veins. When RNOS are abundant or unbalanced by inadequate antioxidant systems, then destruction in the blood vessels can occur.

One of the main pathologies today is atherosclerosis, a disease process where the primary pathology lies in inflammation and damage to the arteries. As new science emerges, the cholesterol theory, which postulated that cholesterol was *the* cause of heart disease, is no longer as strong as the inflammatory and oxidative stress models, because of the ongoing prevalence of cardiovascular disease. Given that over 50 percent of people who experience heart attacks have "normal" cholesterol and LDL (low-density lipoprotein) levels, it has been noted that cholesterol may not be the main cause of heart disease.

Oxidative Stress and Lipid Peroxidation

All of your cell membranes are made of lipids (fats). This enables the cells and their contents to stay together in a liquid environment.

When oxygen radicals interact with your cell membranes, some serious damage can be done to the integrity of the cell membrane, and inevitably the cell itself. Lipid peroxides and malondialdehyde (MDA) are formed when an oxygen radical interacts with the polyunsaturated fats in the cell membrane. Polyunsaturated fats are naturally unstable, compared with saturated fats, as not all of their hydrogen atoms are "saturated" with electrons.

However, a good number of polyunsaturated fats make up your cell membranes. The more oxidative stress and inflammation going on in your body, the more lipid peroxidation occurs, and your cells begin to die.

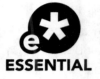

ESSENTIAL

Free radicals produced by your own body can cause damage to tissues and cells. The best way to balance free radical damage is to have a well-supported antioxidant system and a well-adjusted adrenal response. Continually reducing the naturally produced free radicals in your body, with fresh vegetables and fruit, is key to decreasing inflammation and chronic disease.

Free Radicals and Adrenal Fatigue

Interestingly enough, your body will produce ROS and RNOS to stay healthy—or better put: a healthy person will have ROS and RNOS as part of his or her immune/defense mechanism, and that is perfectly normal.

If you are supposed to form free radicals, then what is all the fuss about? Well, these free radicals can be quite dangerous to the body's tissues if they are allowed to exist without limitation. These oxygen radicals damage lipids, proteins (amino acids), sugars, and DNA. So why does something that confers such benefit also have the potential for such destruction, increasing the likelihood of aiding in adrenal fatigue and making it difficult to heal from it? Because these processes can get out of control. There are two main ways this happens:

- Your oxidative stress is higher than in a healthy human being
- The things you need to quiet down the oxidative stress are missing or not well supported

It is really that simple. The balance between oxidation and antioxidants is very well controlled in the body. The problem is when you negatively influence these pathways either because you are exposed to an increased amount of environmental and societal pollutants or because your antioxidant systems are not working as well as they could be due to a poor diet, unhealthy lifestyle, genes that are compromised, or some combination of all three.

Causes of Oxidative Stress

Beyond your body's own ability to produce free radicals, there are numerous chemicals that are either free radicals themselves or create oxidative stress via the body's metabolic and detoxification pathways. Those with advanced adrenal fatigue will have difficulty when exposed to any amount of these chemicals, while those with moderate adrenal fatigue, which is where many individuals fall, will often find that there are certain chemicals on this list that bother you. The goal is to limit as many of these as possible, on an ongoing basis:

- Cigarette smoke
- Ionizing radiation
- Pollution
- Chlorine
- Pesticides
- Antibiotics and hormones from poorly raised animals
- Plastics/bisphenol A (BPA)
- Alcohol
- Pharmaceutical drugs
- A diet full of poor-quality meat and few plants (vegetables)
- Artificial flavorings and dyes (please read ingredient labels)
- Cosmetics and skin cleansers made from petroleum (most "name-brand" products)
- Trauma or injury to the muscle
- Endurance exercise

All of these can contribute to the amount of oxidative stress you have in your body at one time. This is why it is even more important to make sure you are getting everything you need in your daily life to stay healthy.

Get Control of Your Oxidative Stress, Get Control of Your Health

Oxidative stress has been implicated in nearly all diseases, not as a cause of disease but as a major contributor. Numerous researchers have explored how oxidative stress affects health and disease, and a fairly common consensus is that many of our chronic diseases are initiated, or made worse, by

ROS. In the *International Journal of Biomedical Science*, the authors of "Free Radicals, Antioxidants in Disease and Health" researched this matter and included the following chronic and degenerative conditions as largely influenced by ROS:

1. Cancer
2. Cardiovascular diseases: atherosclerosis, myocardial infarction, post-ischemic reperfusion injury (often after a cardiovascular event), stroke
3. Diabetes
4. Osteoarthritis
5. Rheumatoid arthritis and other autoimmune conditions
6. Neurological diseases: Parkinson's disease, Alzheimer's disease
7. Inflammatory bowel disease
8. Atopic (hypersensitivity) diseases: allergies, eczema, asthma
9. Fetal growth restriction and preeclampsia
10. Oxidative stress (accelerates the aging process, too)

Free Radicals and Increased Inflammation

Whether you (want to) believe it or not, an imbalance in ROS is going to lead to inflammation and disease. How that manifests in you can be vastly different from how it manifests in someone else. Disease expression is not just the result of a single cause. Sometimes one thing can be the main instigator of a condition (for instance, cigarette smoke and lung cancer), but in all honesty, most conditions are not that clear-cut.

Ultimately, disease comes from a lifetime of poor dietary choices, poor lifestyle habits, genetics, environmental pollutants, and exposure to chemicals. If you want to get better, you have to correct your diet and lifestyle, reduce your exposure to unnecessary chemicals, antibiotics, and drugs, become nutrient dense (many Americans are calorie dense and nutrient poor), and allow your body to heal. You absolutely have the power to help your body heal and stay well. This book will show you what you can do to increase your body's natural antioxidant systems.

What Is My Body Doing to Counteract Free Radicals?

Fortunately, the body has many mechanisms in place to help get rid of free radicals. This is called the antioxidant defense system. The question you should really be asking is, "How effective is *my* body at getting rid of free radicals?"

Simply put, oxidative stress is out of control when the rate of ROS generation exceeds the capacity of the cell to remove them. The best way to take back control of your health is to improve the health of the cells through a clean diet and lifestyle, so your body is able to purge free radicals. The primary detoxification pathways are a group of organs that help the body get rid of waste, toxins, and chemicals, and include the liver, digestive system, skin, kidneys, and lungs. The process of detoxification is continually happening in your body whether you consciously know it or not. The goal is to have your diet, lifestyle, and habits support these processes so that you can get rid of waste and toxins efficiently and not end up with symptoms or a diagnosed condition.

The body uses the following to turn off ROS:

- Repair processes.
- Compartmentalization.
- Defense "antioxidant" enzymes: your body's own defense antioxidants. They are stronger than most antioxidants you can buy in a health food store. These enzymes include superoxide dismutase (SOD), catalase, glutathione peroxidase, and glutathione reductase.
- Non-enzymatic antioxidants: include **endogenous antioxidants** (from within the body), such as lipoic acid, L-arginine, melatonin, glutathione, coenzyme Q10 (CoQ10), uric acid, bilirubin, metal chelating agents, transferrin, citriulline, taurine; **exogenous antioxidants** (from outside the body) including vitamin C, vitamin E, carotenoids (including vitamin A), omega-3 fatty acids, trace minerals including selenium, manganese, and zinc, and flavonoids.

The exogenous antioxidants obtained from your diet generally assist your own endogenous antioxidant and enzyme systems. This is a primary goal of eating quality food: to nourish biochemical pathways and enzyme systems in the body.

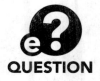

QUESTION

Is it true or false that the body has multiple mechanisms set up to naturally get rid of free radicals and free radical–producing agents?
True, but here is the catch: when these antioxidants donate an electron to help get rid of ROS, they themselves become free radicals, and you need to fuel your antioxidant pathways. Therefore, it is so important to always be providing the body with the antioxidants, vitamins, minerals, and nutrients it uses to either make or support the antioxidant defense system.

Oxidative Stress, Cortisol, and Neurodegenerative Disease

A fair amount of research these days is looking at how ROS affects neurological health. With untreatable conditions on the rise including Parkinson's disease, Alzheimer's disease, amyotrophic lateral sclerosis (ALS), and multiple sclerosis (MS), one has to wonder if there is something in daily life causing these chronic degenerative diseases, or at the very least contributing to such devastating conditions.

Neurological conditions are often very serious, and end up causing a whole lot of other symptoms in the body because the nervous system affects every system. Figuring out why there is an increase in these neurodegenerative conditions is a step in the right direction. The next step, of course, would be to ask why neurodegeneration is happening in the brain, and what exactly ROS has to do with it.

Fortunately, researchers have found that metals are more common in the brains of persons suffering from these neurodegenerative diseases. Zinc, copper, iron—all normal metals used by the body in biochemical reactions, which also support the production of ROS.

Parkinson's disease has pathological findings of copper and iron, which interact with dopamine, a chelating agent itself. When something is a chelator, it means that some of its molecules can form several bonds to a single metal ion. It is noted that in individuals with genetic tendencies toward increased activity of dopamine, reactions between dopamine and metals create hydrogen peroxide. The body's way of getting rid of hydrogen peroxide, of course, is to make water and a hydroxyl radical. This free radical, without enough antioxidant opposition, is damaging, especially in the brain.

In Alzheimer's disease, plaque formation is one of the main pathological findings. This occurs from the chelation of amyloid-beta peptide by "transition" metals: zinc, copper, and iron. Transition metals readily move between a reduced and oxidized state, taking and donating electrons. These metals bind to the amyloid-beta peptide, and the reaction produces hydrogen peroxide (H_2O_2).

Now if you circle back to how the body gets rid of H_2O_2, you may recall that it will produce a hydroxyl radical. Therefore, the next logical scientific question would be, "If you had sufficient antioxidant pathways supported, would you be able to prevent this damage from occurring?" Only time and research will tell.

In addition to ROS, a key hallmark of Alzheimer's is insulin receptor desensitization in the brain and glucose accumulation. Most of these discoveries have only been made in autopsies once patients are deceased, because evaluating someone's brain while they are alive is not an easy practice. One of cortisol's main roles, as you know by now, is to increase blood sugar in the body, including in the brain. Some researchers even postulate that Alzheimer's may be a type of diabetes, uniquely different from DM1 and DM2.

While this may all seem scary, one thing is for sure: ROS is implicated in nearly all disease, and in order to heal your body, heal your adrenals, and support long-term health, you must reduce oxidative stress and inflammation. With growing numbers of individuals developing neurodegenerative conditions, assessing where you may be experiencing excessive ROS in conjunction with diagnosing and properly treating your adrenal fatigue seems like logical preventative steps in helping to reduce disease development and progression, especially in the brain.

Simply Start with This

What you can start doing today to get your inflammation under control is not difficult. Given that antioxidants are well documented as necessary for recycling and reducing free radicals, one sure way to beat oxidative stress and inflammation from causing you harm is to include more antioxidants in your diet. This is super easy. All of your fruits and vegetables have varying degrees of antioxidants in them. Think mostly dark fruits, green leafy plants, and the rainbow of vegetables when looking to add to your diet.

❑ **Dark berries:** blueberry, blackberry, boysenberry, raspberry, strawberry, cherry, huckleberry, goji berry
❑ **Dark vegetables:** collards, spinach, kale, mustard, arugula, chard, bok choy, broccoli, Brussels sprouts, beets
❑ **Other antioxidant-rich foods:** plums, grapes, nectarines, butternut squash, and peaches

Here's one quick way to increase your intake: add two more servings (1 cup raw or ½ cup cooked) of an antioxidant-rich fruit and antioxidant-rich vegetable into your diet today.

CHAPTER 4

Do I Have Adrenal Fatigue?

Taking the time to find out whether you have adrenal fatigue, and to what severity, is now more and more common among healthcare practitioners. Once an accurate assessment and diagnosis is made, restoring health to the adrenal glands can be accomplished. Understanding where your adrenal gland function is on the scale of adrenal fatigue will help you know what support is needed to heal your body. In the long run, knowing how your stress response affects your health will empower you to understand how to positively influence your stress response. As the conventional medical model catches up with the science, more professionals will choose accurate testing, a comprehensive approach to treatment, and the restoration of health over symptom management.

Defining Adrenal Fatigue (Hypoadrenia)

Hypoadrenia literally means "lower" (*hypo*), "related to the adrenals" (*adrenia*): a deficiency of the adrenal glands. The adrenal glands are constantly secreting small amounts of steroid hormones through the natural circadian rhythm, the "sleep-wake" cycle, and in response to a stressor. The adrenal glands do this in a very controlled manner, through negative feedback loops set up with the brain and the central nervous system.

During the sleep-wake cycle, there is an abundance of cortisol output, roughly 50 percent of total cortisol, beginning around 6 A.M. and peaking at 8 A.M., with the lowest cortisol output being around midnight. On the other hand, as the body responds to a stressor, whether physical, emotional, or psychological, cortisol output increases. Once the stress has occurred the body responds, and eventually the feedback loops let cortisol, and other chemical messengers, go back to baseline.

Simply put, hypoadrenia results when a complex physiological response to one stress after another is experienced day in and day out, without appropriate restoration of health in between each stress. This heightened and ongoing response to stress eventually creates problems with homeostasis in the normal circadian rhythm, resulting in a decreased output of cortisol.

FACT

Focusing on balancing the sleep-wake cycle, the circadian rhythm, by supporting daytime wakefulness, nighttime restorative sleep, and a better response to stress throughout the day will help you heal the adrenals and promote more energy, better sleep, and better long-term health.

For instance, if you experience increased stress later in the day (driving home from work, making dinner for your family, getting the kids to bed and finally winding down yourself), you are pushing your circadian rhythm too hard later in the day. While these tasks are all necessary and you probably can't change them, your response to the events/stressors could be causing your body to elevate cortisol between the hours of 5–9 P.M., making it very difficult for your body to naturally fall into the normal sleep-wake cycle of having a lowered cortisol at this time, when you normally should, right before you go to bed.

If this scenario is common, eventually you would expect to see a high salivary cortisol reading right before bed in laboratory testing, leading to a concurrent disruption in morning time and afternoon cortisol rhythms. You would eventually start experiencing such symptoms as daytime exhaustion/ fatigue and difficulty sleeping or insomnia at night.

The Conventional Model of Hypoadrenia

In the conventional medical model, hypoadrenia only occurs when one develops Addison's disease. This is a severe condition and is relatively rare, often being the result of autoimmune disease. An individual with Addison's will need to take cortisol for the entirety of her life, because the adrenal glands just don't produce enough of it. You couldn't live without sufficient levels of cortisol.

Why Do I Feel So Good?

On the road to adrenal fatigue you will actually move toward hyper-adrenia or "higher adrenal gland" function first. Many who experience this don't even know they are in a heightened state of cortisol output. In fact, individuals who work the 60-hour workweek (and love it) get a rush from it. These people are in the adrenal overdrive state. Most people live in this state into their early twenties and will be able to do things such as pull all-nighters or push themselves to do more and more, rebounding fairly easily. The adrenal "bank account" (stay tuned for more on that) is fairly full, or at least full enough, that for every withdrawal you make, you still have enough energy to stay healthy.

How You Got to Hypoadrenia/Adrenal Fatigue

Eventually the elevated cortisol state will give way to a lowered state of adrenal gland function, showing up in various symptoms. This is when it is more common for an individual to seek help. Symptoms such as fatigue, inability to focus, daytime exhaustion, poor sleep, and so on, become more prevalent. Just remember, if you are one of those individuals with a constantly on-the-go lifestyle and you are feeling good (maybe the only symptom you have is little sleep, which you equate to being fine because you get more done), eventually you will push yourself too far, and the pendulum will swing the other way, into true adrenal fatigue.

What Causes Hypoadrenia?

Hypoadrenia is the underfunctioning of the adrenal glands due to prolonged and/or intense stress. The stress can be physical, mental/psychological, emotional, infectious, genetic, and environmental, or some combination of these. The type of stress doesn't matter, but your response to the stressor does. Remember, your body responds the same way no matter what source the stress is from. Once your body and mind perceive a stress, the endocrine and nervous system respond accordingly.

The Adrenal Bank Account

Adrenal fatigue ultimately happens when the body's ability to cope with the stressors is not strong enough to recuperate after the stressor. Again, if this is equated to a savings account, you want to have more deposits than withdrawals. A deposit would be 7–8 hours of quality sleep, good dietary choices, appropriate exercise, fresh air, daily sunlight, and so on. Withdrawals are all of the stress responses—the time you push yourself to stay up late to finish a project or wake up early to get things done before the kids are up, taking care of others without taking care of yourself, consuming caffeine to wake up, consuming alcohol or sleep aids to fall asleep, and so on.

Over time, as the withdrawals become more abundant than the deposits, you eventually fall into the negative. Those with a strong mental state may even push themselves to "go further" even once the bank account is empty, ultimately causing a more severe burnout once the body just can't push anymore. At that point, systemic symptoms develop. If the adrenal glands are treated, many of the systemic symptoms would also heal.

Three Most Common Causes of Hypoadrenia

Although adrenal fatigue can be caused by many factors, the following are the most commonly seen causes of adrenal fatigue:

❑ Grief, loss, or death of a loved one
❑ Inflammation that is ongoing and uncontrolled
❑ Poor dietary and lifestyle choices

Hypoadrenia can develop from one major stressor or multiple small stressors. Most commonly, a person experiences many small and medium stressors throughout life, and then a major event sends his body into adrenal fatigue. Another person may experience one large trauma, and that is enough to send her body into complete adrenal exhaustion. The one common theme that leaves most people unable to respond appropriately to multiple stressors or a major stressor is poor dietary and lifestyle choices.

Adrenal Fatigue as a Spectrum

Adrenal fatigue follows a curve. There is the normal stress response on the far left, when you incur a stress and respond appropriately, then your body returns to a normal, healthy homeostasis. As you incur more stressors without appropriate recovery between them, you most likely move into hyperadrenia, or overwork of adrenal gland function, where excess cortisol/steroid hormone output occurs continually. This causes the "normal" line of cortisol output to spike. During this phase, a lot more oxidative stress will occur in the adrenal glands because of the sheer amount of hormones that are being made. Remember that when cells are busy, they burn through oxygen to fuel the mitochondria and produce ATP, the energy of the cells.

As you continue on the path of adrenal gland dysfunction, eventually the cortisol line falls, well below normal, and this is where complete burnout or exhaustion exists. This is what most refer to as hypoadrenia or adrenal fatigue. There is global inflammation and systemic symptoms caused by long-term oxidative stress during the hyper state, and now there is a lack of cortisone, cortisol's precursor to respond to the body's ongoing inflammatory burden.

Within the curve, there are multiple steps before one gets to adrenal fatigue, including a spike of cortisol output that puts you into hyperadrenia, *not* characteristic of "adrenal burnout." This is why it is so important to really have an individualized approach to your treatment. Just taking whatever is out there for adrenal support may not be exactly what you need. Knowing where you fall on the spectrum of adrenal fatigue is the best first step to help you get the most specific treatment for you, and to really help your adrenal/endocrine system heal.

QUESTION

Are the adrenal glands really able to recover after stress?
Yes, the adrenal glands are designed to respond to stressors and return to homeostasis once the stress is over. However, key nutrients, including vitamins C and B$_5$, cholesterol, and essential fatty acids and lifestyle habits will make it easier for your adrenal glands to bounce back after a life stress.

The adrenal curve will most likely move as a result of the following: repeated stressors, death of a loved one (human or animal), loss of work, infection (bronchitis or pneumonia), allergies, lack of sleep or lack of restorative sleep, poor dietary choices, lack of exercise or excessive exercise, toxins/pollutants, fear, caffeine, alcohol, sugar, no down time, no enjoyment in life, depression, anxiety, financial pressures, drugs, stress from partner or spouse, negative beliefs, nicotine, pesticides, etc.

How Adrenal Fatigue Progresses

When looking to properly evaluate adrenal fatigue, the best way to assess the extent of your condition is to use your symptoms combined with laboratory findings to place your progress on a scale.

By placing adrenal fatigue on a spectrum, it becomes clearer how your body is currently responding to stress: properly, excessively, or inadequately. This information will allow treatment to get even more specific. For instance, if you have an exaggerated stress response, you would not benefit from an herb that is stimulating to the adrenal system. In fact, that could cause adverse side effects. Let's take a look at how to classify the different stages of adrenal fatigue.

The Maladaptive Stress Syndrome (MSS)

Following is one of the most common ways to categorize adrenal fatigue, based on the work of Hans Selye, and further substantiated by the current medical practices around adrenal fatigue.

MSS Stage/Type 0

This stage includes normal function of the adrenal glands. Your body normally swings between "high" cortisol for wake periods and "low" cortisol for sleep periods, all within the normal range of cortisol. The stress response is not a main factor of evaluation, as this stage mostly deals with being awake, alert, and oriented, complemented by being in a deep restorative sleep overnight. This is the foundation from which a healthy adrenal response operates.

MSS Stage/Type 1

The alarm state of adrenal gland function is found in this stage, and is associated with a higher than normal release of cortisol and epinephrine for the time of day. This is the stereotypical fight-or-flight alarm that goes off in the body. As long as appropriate lifestyle habits, diet, and nourishment are maintained, the individual can return to MSS0 regularly. Rarely do people live in a "healthier" state than MSS1 because of the common on-the-go lifestyle. A normal cortisol response is roughly 9.2mg/day for the average unstressed adult, but can vary from 8–25mg/day with increasing stress.

MSS Stage/Type 2

This phase is known as the suppression stage of adrenal exhaustion. Findings include increased amounts of cortisol and neurotransmitters such as epinephrine and norepinephrine. Cortisol will cause hyperglycemia, the breakdown of skeletal muscle, inflammation modulation, a negative influence on insulin receptors to prevent storage of glucose, and a whole host of other physiological reactions at an accelerated rate.

Increased oxidative stress is common as the adrenals are required to make more steroid hormones: glucocorticoids, mineralocorticoids, and sex hormones. This results in local and systemic inflammation, requiring more cortisol. Blood pressure becomes elevated, and the kidneys must process more minerals. Sex hormones (estrogen and testosterone) become unbalanced as DHEA (dehydroepiandrosterone-sulfate) production is shunted toward progesterone and cortisol; progesterone decreases as it is a precursor to cortisol creation; androgen production increases, causing a potential increase in hair growth, as well as excess estrogen or testosterone; digestion becomes poor, causing symptoms from reflux and bloating to gastritis and constipation; anxiety and depression increase from the higher levels of cortisol and a constantly "on" adrenal response; and the thyroid has to work harder to provide the body with thyroid hormones (T4/T3) to support increased metabolic pathways. Systemic symptoms and conditions are common.

MSS Stage/Type 3

Exhaustion of the HPA axis is the main finding in this phase. This is when you are unable to produce adequate cortisol levels. There may be abnormal fluctuations in cortisol output, less in the morning and more at night, but the overall daily total amount is decreased.

Individuals who fall within MSS3 will experience conditions such as chronic fatigue, fibromyalgia, hypotension, chemical sensitivity, odor sensitivity, atypical depression or apathy, poor resistance to infection, etc. During this stage, hypoglycemia is common and symptoms of hypoglycemia become more apparent to the individual (light-headedness, dizziness, shakiness, irritability, etc.). The body will attempt to compensate for the lack of cortisol with surges of epinephrine. Therefore, anxiety and irritability, confusion, and lack of focus are common symptoms in the exhaustion phase.

Determining the Phases

The stages defined by the maladaptive stress syndrome allow you to assess where your adrenal gland function lands, giving you the information you need to find an appropriate treatment plan. You will be able to assess what phase you are in by using laboratory testing along with current symptoms and a well-documented case history. It is important to note that you can be in between stages. Many people fall somewhere between stage 2 and stage 3. Those with stage 3 are often individuals who have experienced chronic conditions most of their life, or are diagnosed with a condition such as chronic fatigue syndrome, fibromyalgia, multiple chemical sensitivity, and so forth. For those of you who are in stage three, additional considerations may be warranted depending on how other hormones in your body respond to depressed cortisol.

Two Different Types of Burnout

Adrenal fatigue is sometimes referred to as adrenal burnout, and yet adrenal burnout is a more appropriate term for the end stage of adrenal fatigue. Adrenal fatigue really just means that the adrenal glands can no longer respond the way they normally should be able to, by appropriately putting out hormones and neurotransmitters in response to stress. So essentially, the adrenal glands have "burned" themselves out. This equates to stage 3 of the maladaptive stress syndrome.

To make matters even more complicated, there are two different responses your body could have physiologically when adrenal burnout happens. It is not clear why individuals react so uniquely—possibly from genetics or the type of stress that initiated the adrenal burnout—but one thing is clear: individuals can become either serotonin-depleted or dopamine-depleted when burnout is near. Dopamine primarily functions as part of the reward driven parts of the brain, whereas serotonin affects the brain and the body including appetite, sexual urges, sleep, memory, learning, and more.

In the journal *Neuropsychobiology*, the article "The Psychobiology of Burnout" reported on the hypothesis that there are unique differences in specific hormones corresponding with adrenal burnout symptoms, including cortisol, prolactin, oxytocin, and ACTH. The authors were attempting to understand whether a more specific treatment routine could be given to those suffering from the condition, as treatment with cortisol provides mixed results in improving adrenal burnout.

ESSENTIAL

Your adrenal glands work hard for you and require that you nourish and take care of them on a daily basis. One thing you can do today is to make sure you are drinking adequate amounts of water, which supports healthy skin, hair, blood pressure, and adrenal glands. The goal is to drink one-half your body weight in ounces daily. Get started today!

In the study reported in that article, individuals with severe symptoms of adrenal burnout, prolactin levels were either high or low. Prolactin has over 300 functions in the body, including suppression of dopamine. In individuals whose prolactin levels were low, they also experienced low serotonin and tended to have lower oxytocin levels along with low attachment scores, as oxytocin is released when one feels loved. In those individuals with high prolactin corresponding to adrenal burnout symptoms, dopamine was low, and treatment with exogenous cortisol caused a resulting decrease in prolactin and fatigue, while increasing vigor, allowing dopamine levels to return to normal.

What this research demonstrates is that when it comes to adrenal burnout, each person may need a slightly different treatment plan to help the adrenal glands heal. Thus, it is helpful not only to differentiate where you fall within the maladaptive stress syndrome staging but also to measure certain hormones within the body. Doing so is especially beneficial for those who truly are in adrenal burnout/MSS Stage 3.

For example, cortisol supplementation is a common prescription in those individuals with severe adrenal fatigue. Whether this is a smart prescription for you and whether you will respond positively could rest on whether you have low serotonergic function or low dopaminergic function.

Common Symptoms of Adrenal Fatigue

Adrenal fatigue, as a diagnosis, presents with many varied symptoms, and yet there is an underlying theme to the symptoms that comes from the adrenals themselves. While those with adrenal fatigue will have symptoms in multiple systems (for instance, you may have high blood pressure, blood sugar issues, premenstrual syndrome, and anxiety), there are specific symptoms of hypoadrenia that simultaneously begin to become noticeable.

While you could look at these as separate symptoms coming from various systems and treat them individually, a better treatment response is to look at them as interconnected issues. The following is a common list of symptoms coming from the adrenal glands, which often present in addition to symptoms from a heightened stress response:

- Difficulty getting up in the morning
- Strong salt cravings or strong sugar cravings (usually one or the other, not both)
- Daytime fatigue that is not relieved by any amount of sleep
- Low energy and lots of effort to complete daily tasks
- Lowered or no libido
- Difficulty handling stress, decreased productivity
- Increased emotional symptoms including anxiety, irritability, depression

- Trouble recovering from illnesses, chronic infections
- Lightheadedness when standing quickly, ongoing ringing in the ears
- Worsening of symptoms if meals are skipped
- Lack of focus, "brain fog," memory loss
- Exhaustion in the morning, crashes in the early afternoon, energy bursts after dinner at night

These symptoms develop because your adrenal glands are no longer able to cope with the stressors you impose upon them. These are true symptoms of adrenal gland dysfunction, and understanding what your specific diagnosis is in the maladaptive stress syndrome (MSS) staging will help you know what specific treatments you need to heal your adrenal glands and your health.

What All Adrenal Glands Need

Normally, the adrenal glands restore balance in between each stressor. This means that all the hormones involved in the stress reaction go back to a baseline value. The hypothalamus stops releasing corticotrophin-releasing hormone (CRH), the pituitary stops releasing adrenocorticotropic hormone (ACTH), and the adrenals reduce their release of cortisol. If you are like most people, you aren't letting your adrenal glands heal after each stressor. Instead you experience a stressor, recover enough to continue to go about your day (maybe), and then you experience another stressor.

Now, suppose you just changed your diet and lifestyle habits to be more supportive of your adrenal gland health. Suppose you had the right lifestyle habits to support a healthy adrenal response; wouldn't you assume you would be much better off, and have a better chance at recovering from stressors and bouncing back? Imagine that every day you did a lot more to fill up your adrenal bank account instead of completely depleting it. Then when you wanted to make a withdrawal, you had plenty of reserves, so that your balance wouldn't be at zero—it wouldn't even be close.

This way, you are living a preventative lifestyle that feeds your adrenal gland health and your whole body's health. But what does that look like? In order to restore function to the adrenal glands, a complex combination of diet, lifestyle factors, circadian rhythm normalization, nutrients, and herbs appropriate to your constitution and level of adrenal fatigue is necessary. For instance, two well-known herbs for the adrenal glands are the ginsengs. Asian ginseng (*Panax ginseng*) is much more stimulating than American ginseng (*Panax quinquefolius*), so you may become overstimulated by the Asian ginseng.

Prior to supplementing with the newest adrenal supplement, energy drink, or focus powder, it is best to remember that your symptoms are a reflection of your stress response, your adrenal health, and ultimately where you lie on the scale of adrenal fatigue. Taking inventory of your lifestyle and uncovering what you are doing on a daily basis to either support your adrenal glands or potentially hurt them is key in being able to turn yourself around on the path, and begin walking on the road of adrenal gland health.

CHAPTER 5

Signs and Symptoms of Adrenal Fatigue

Fortunately, the medical community and the population at large are getting better at recognizing the signs and symptoms of adrenal fatigue. When you try to treat symptoms in various areas of your body without addressing your adrenal glands, you are not going to get very far; at best, you will be able to manage your symptoms by taking a pill, whether pharmaceutical or natural. Every system in your body relies on a healthy adrenal gland system, so if you have a symptom somewhere in your body, it likely has some part of adrenal gland dysfunction contributing to it. While symptom expression is unique to each individual based on genetics, upbringing, diet, environment, and social influence, this chapter is devoted to the more common symptoms connecting back to a poorly functioning adrenal gland system. These symptoms result from the adrenal gland working too hard for too long.

Fatigue, Chronic Fatigue, and Insomnia

Fatigue is a word that is commonly used today to describe feeling tired. The way it presents itself can be different to each person. You may experience fatigue in the beginning of the day, you may experience it in the middle of the day, or you may crash at night. Whether it comes from a busy lifestyle, a lack of enthusiasm about daily life, an adrenal gland bank account being empty, or most likely some combination of all of these, one thing is for sure: most people experience fatigue at some point in life.

ALERT

To heal the adrenal glands, one of the most important things you will need to do is regulate your sleep-wake cycle. This means that morning time needs to be focused on stimulating the body through exercise or getting outside, maybe even both! Natural light does wonders for suppressing melatonin production from the pineal gland. Suppressing melatonin in the morning will help your body wake up.

Why You're Fatigued

You may remember the exact moment in life when you felt like a switch turned off and the fatigue began, or you may never remember a day when you weren't tired. The truth of the matter is, you, like many, may be living an overly stressed lifestyle and your adrenal glands are having a hard time keeping up with the pace.

This overloaded lifestyle is problematic because your stress response and adrenal system respond to one stressor after another: kids, spouse, finances, boss, employee, etc. You may not even be conscious of what is physically happening in your body under all these stressors, and you aren't recovering between all the chores on your to-do list. Plus you don't get a chance to do the things that support health in your adrenal glands. And most importantly, you aren't allowing yourself to enjoy life.

Now, maybe for you, things don't look quite that repetitive. Maybe at this point in your life, you have learned that a good breakfast can get you a long way, or that taking a walk in the afternoon is much better than a second or third cup of coffee. However, you still experience fatigue or other symptoms that make you wonder whether your adrenal glands are functioning at their optimal level.

Chronic Fatigue Syndrome

Chronic fatigue syndrome (CFS) is a complex condition, often with no apparent underlying medical diagnosis. The classical symptoms are extreme fatigue and fatigue that does not get better with rest, no matter how much rest. Often, there is something that triggers CFS in an individual who already has a weakened constitution and/or a compromised adrenal response system. These triggers can include: viral infections, immunological issues, psychological stress, and hormonal imbalance. The adrenal system is sometimes so exhausted that it can't even respond in a normal fashion to acute stressors, leaving the individual virtually "defenseless" and exhausted. These individuals tend to experience more illnesses, inability to recover from illnesses, and other systemic symptoms such as brain fog/fatigue, sensitivity to chemicals, and so on.

Insomnia from Stress

Sleep issues are one of the most common symptoms reported in modern times. A huge variety of pharmaceutical medications are used for sleep disorders, including central nervous system depressants, melatonin receptor agonists, anxiolytics, hypnotics, antidepressants, benzodiazepines, and so forth. If you aren't on a medication to help you sleep, chances are you may be using other substances such as alcohol to help you calm down your nervous system and adrenal system in order to get to sleep. Living in a pick-me-up world makes it extremely hard to get the body to naturally calm down. What happens then is even though you are exhausted at the end of the day, your body can't relax enough to fully sleep. This means your body is unable to fully repair and restore every night while in deep sleep.

ESSENTIAL

One main contributor to poor sleep quality is the health of your adrenal glands. When you push yourself during the daytime, eventually you burn out your adrenals, which can cause a disturbance to the natural rhythm of the sleep-wake cycle. Eventually cortisol spikes are seen prior to bed, around 10 P.M., or in the middle of the night between 1–3 A.M., causing insomnia.

THERE ARE THREE MAIN REASONS ONE HAS FATIGUE AND/OR SLEEP ISSUES:

- You are not living the life of your dreams, or you have decided to just live "the autopilot life"
- The sleep-wake cycle is disrupted
- Your adrenal bank account is empty

In order to truly heal your adrenal glands and get rid of fatigue, you must support a healthy adrenal gland reserve by filling up your bank account with deposits every day, you must regulate your sleep-wake cycle, and you must start to live the life that you envision yourself living, not necessarily the one you are currently living. You have a reason and purpose for being here and uncovering this purpose will help your body, mind, and spirit heal.

Your adrenal glands thrive on a well-supported sleep-wake cycle. What you may not realize is that your energy level during the day is a direct reflection of your sleep state, and your ability to get into a deep sleep is a reflection of your energy levels during the day.

Many people end up having low cortisol during the day because of living a very busy lifestyle without making sure the adrenal bank account is filled up daily. This often results in an increase in cortisol at night. This may be an actual increase in cortisol overnight, or it may be a relative elevation of cortisol at night compared to daytime cortisol being so low. Whether you have sleep difficulties because you are exhausted during the day or because your cortisol is elevated at night (or likely both), getting a good night's sleep will be one of the primary tasks in restoring health to the adrenal glands.

While sleep is important, and getting a good night's sleep with medications is better than a poor night's sleep without medications, eventually you'll need to come off the medications in order to regulate your sleep-wake cycle and heal your adrenal glands. There are numerous other ways to regulate your sleep-wake cycle that you will see in the coming chapters. As for living a fulfilled life and filling up your adrenal bank account, just know that healing is a journey, and in this book you will learn what it takes to keep yourself moving forward on the path of healing.

Blood Pressure and Cardiovascular Changes

Both cortisol and the neurotransmitters released from the adrenal glands have specific effects on the cardiovascular system. For instance, epinephrine, which is released immediately when an acute stressor is experienced, increases heart rate and blood pressure. As the body works to maintain the stress response, cortisol will support the initial role of epinephrine to maintain an elevated blood pressure to get blood around the body more quickly so that tissues can have a ready supply of oxygen (blood carries oxygen around the body). This is great in an acute response when you need to react immediately to a threat, but over the long term, constant stimulation of the cardiovascular system by both epinephrine and cortisol has deleterious effects.

On top of increasing heart rate, these hormones, mediated by the nervous system, cause vasoconstriction of the blood vessels, thereby increasing blood pressure. There is good reason to want to lower blood pressure if it is continually elevated. Studies show that hypertension leads to heart attacks, ischemic strokes, dementia, heart failure, and all-cause mortality. The normal blood pressure reading of $120/80$ is hard to maintain when cortisol and epinephrine are continually being released into the body at sustained and elevated levels.

Naturally, there is great variability to blood pressure and heart rate in any individual over time. This is actually quite healthy. Individuals with reduced heart rate variability are often more likely to develop cardiovascular-related conditions and are less likely to recover after a heart attack. So you want to be able to have good heart rate variability without elevated blood pressure.

Amazingly enough, 95 percent of cases of hypertension, or what is considered "essential" hypertension, is from unknown causes. This type of hypertension is also referred to as primary or idiopathic. Given that there are well over 100 different pharmaceuticals to treat hypertension, it is amazing that the cause of primary hypertension has not been identified. Rather, the medical community suffices at treating the problem, but not identifying and treating the root cause.

The most common causes for elevated blood pressure are physical stress, "white coat hypertension (when you see the doctor)," work strain, environmental causes such as exposure to toxins and chemicals, poor dietary choices, social issues, race/ethnicity, and emotional distress. It may be more appropriate to look at hypertension as a state of imbalance rather than a condition in and of itself, and only look at it as a diagnosis when the cause can be traced back to an anatomical or physiological change to the body. Examples of such causes of high blood pressure include coarctation of the aorta, unilateral renal disease, pheochromocytoma, or primary aldosteronism.

If primary hypertension has no "known" cause, but only things that may "contribute," then maybe the next best first step to treating high blood pressure is to remove a contributing factor such as exposure to cigarette smoke or replace what is missing, such as electrolytes from vegetables in your diet. For instance, physical and emotional stress both contribute to elevated blood pressure. So why not learn how to balance your stress response with specific therapies such as meditation, acupuncture, massage, or exercise? Better yet, do a combination of any of those. Then throw in some other modifications from "contributors," such as reducing intake of processed foods that contain a lot of sodium, food additives, and artificial colorings, increasing consumption of fresh vegetables, reducing caffeine intake, and getting adequate exercise.

Anxiety, Irritability, Depression

Mental and emotional symptoms from an exhausted adrenal response are common. Oftentimes an individual is predisposed to react a certain way to the world. Maybe you are the classic worrier who always thinks about what could go wrong, what will go wrong, or what has gone wrong. This often brings about feelings of anxiety or helplessness.

On the other hand, you may be the type of person who becomes extremely irritable and defensive when you are in an acute stressful situation. Beyond making it difficult to communicate, irritability can cause lack of focus and shortsightedness on tasks that need attention to detail. If this is your fallback emotion, adrenal fatigue can make this more pronounced.

The third most common emotional reaction to stressful situations is depression, withdrawal, or apathy. Adrenal fatigue can make any of these three types of reactions more pronounced, and harder to manage. While your constitution may have a normal disposition to one of the three, adrenal fatigue can make the symptoms stronger and more difficult to balance in your day-to-day life.

Anxiety and Adrenal Fatigue

Anxiety is a common feeling most everyone will experience at some point in life. The way you experience anxiety is often unique to you, manifesting as increased heart rate, difficulty breathing, shallow breathing, tightening of the digestive system experienced as indigestion or lack of appetite, racing thoughts, a scattered mind, overly emotionally reactive, tightening of the chest, inability to sit still, and so on.

One of the biggest things for those who suffer from anxiety is realizing that they cannot control everything. Unless you realize that many things are out of your control, *and learn to be okay with that*, anxiety is harder to manage. If you suffer from anxiety, it is important to identify what triggers the anxiety and remove it or avoid it if at all possible. You will need to learn some techniques required to keep your mental and emotional state in better balance, while healing your adrenal system. Adrenal glands that are not well nourished will push you into your imbalanced states more frequently and severely. Often with conditions such as anxiety, you can begin to work on your sleep-wake cycle, improving mindfulness practices, eating better, removing sugar and caffeine, and you will see your anxiety begin to decrease.

Irritability and Adrenal Fatigue

Irritability is a feeling that often stems from not being able to do something. This state of feeling commonly comes from unaccomplished goals, inability to finish a task to completion prior to a deadline, or having unrealistic deadlines. If you are someone who often feels irritable or easily loses control of your temper, most likely your adrenal gland system is negatively impacted.

Now, some individuals also experience simultaneous challenges with emotional expression, often stemming from childhood. This can also contribute to feelings of irritability. Whether you experience irritability because this is your constitution or because you were not well supported emotionally as a child, when your adrenal system is fatigued, you revert to more immature states.

Irritability relates to the feel-good hormones, dopamine and serotonin, which can be inappropriately released or abundantly released, leading to issues with overexcitability in the central nervous system. This can happen through many variables, including poor diet, high sugar intake, low-quality fat and protein intake, addiction to drugs and/or alcohol, stimulants, poor clearance of hormones through the liver, and so on.

Depression, Apathy, Withdrawal, and Adrenal Fatigue

Apathy and depression are other emotions you may experience when you have adrenal fatigue. This depends a lot on your predisposing factors. You may be more likely to experience depression if you feel that you are alone in the world, have no one to reach out to, or are unfulfilled in life, such as being at a dead-end job.

Feelings of helplessness may result when the previously mentioned situations are not supported. For example, if you go to your job day in and day out only because you need money to pay your bills, yet the work environment is mundane and understimulating, negative, and just plain joyless, you are less likely to be able to correct the depression or apathy because you're not remedying the underlying cause.

It is common for individuals to withdraw from life, both as a result of life's situations and in response to a declining function of the adrenal system. Maybe it is time for you to change your job, but you're not ready to go there. At the very least you can begin to support and heal your adrenal system so that the daily grind of a job you don't care for is less detrimental to your overall well-being.

Weight Changes and Food Cravings

Managing weight is one of the most difficult challenges these days for many. In fact, obesity is one of the most prevalent conditions in the Western world, and obesity puts you at risk for a whole host of issues including heart disease, diabetes, joint degradation and musculoskeletal issues, increased body burden of environmental toxins (fat stores toxins), and shortened life expectancy. It is indeed healthy to want to lose weight if you are carrying around some extra pounds, especially if it is in the midsection.

Weight Around the Abdomen

If you are struggling with weight gain around the abdomen, this is one of the classic signs of adrenal gland dysfunction. When you ask your body to continually release cortisol through an unregulated adrenal response, you are triggering one of the main functions of cortisol: redepositing fat from the peripheral tissues to the abdominal area. Cortisol mobilizes triglycerides from storage and deposits them into the visceral adipocytes (fat cells). Visceral fat is under the muscle, deep in the abdomen. The primary goal of this is for "organ protection." The problem is, this type of fat is not good for long-term health. In fact, visceral fat increases your preponderance to conditions such as heart disease and diabetes (notice the running theme here).

QUESTION

Why is it so hard to lose weight?
Many people struggle with weight challenges. Often weight loss can be challenging for a number of reasons, including poor dietary choices, yo-yo dieting, and lack of a regular exercise routine. Other major factors affecting your ability to lose weight are your cortisol levels and your stress response. Elevated cortisol causes fat storage and cuts off fuel burning. So if you struggle with weight loss, make sure your adrenal glands have the right support to really get the results you want.

Cortisol also increases the maturation rate of adipocytes through enzyme control, which converts cortisone into cortisol, via the enzyme 11-beta hydroxysteroid dehydrogenase. Strangely, cortisol regulates its own production by increasing the amount of cortisone being converted to cortisol by stimulating that enzyme. Visceral fat not only has more receptors for cortisol, which means greater utilization of cortisol, but may potentially have more of the enzyme to convert cortisone to cortisol.

No wonder it's so hard to lose that weight! It is hard, for sure, but not impossible. In fact, commitment to regular cardiovascular exercise, not too much, is one of the best ways to shed abdominal fat. The next best thing to do is to get a better handle on your stress response and use strategies such as your diet, herbs, and natural therapies to support the adrenal glands and improve lipolysis (breakdown of fat). By incorporating these basic approaches into your daily lifestyle, you will conquer your abdominal fat and in a few months you will see that stubborn fat shed away.

Craving Control

Cravings can be difficult for some people to get ahold of; sometimes it is a matter of willpower, but often it is about getting control of chemical reactions in your body by better balancing your blood sugar and energy reserves. Cravings are one of the most important aspects of your diet to manage, because they can often be the thing that continually sabotages you and brings you back to the starting place of weight loss.

When you have a healthy appetite and are not plagued by cravings, you feel satiated after your meal. For instance, say you bring your lunch and you have a mixed field green salad with vegetables on it and some sliced roasted chicken with a nice homemade dressing of olive oil and balsamic vinaigrette. Now normally you would feel content and full after a meal like this if your appetite and blood sugar were in better balance, but because your body is fueled by too much sugar, your brain will tell your body that it needs more fuel.

If you often rely on sugar or simple carbohydrates to fuel yourself, you will crave those simple sugars, because your brain and body know it is a "quick fix" to blood sugar dips. This isn't sustainable fuel, and so you will need more and more (and more), and your body will tell you it wants those bad foods. Cravings are part mental and part biochemical. Once you change your diet and get better control of your blood sugar and glycemic index, you will be able to curb the cravings for good!

Effect of Stress on the Immune System

One of the main roles of cortisol is to quiet down the inflammatory response in the immune system. This is why cortisone or corticosteroids are commonly prescribed when the immune system is out of hand. Quieting it down will at least provide you with some (temporary) relief.

Cortisol and its precursor, cortisone, are the strongest anti-inflammatory chemicals your body makes. They are so strong that medicine has replicated them and uses them to your advantage. The only issue is that it doesn't really solve the underlying problem of why the inflammatory process is out of control. It only suppresses the immune system, which is great in some instances but not many. The immune system is an amazingly mysterious and largely unknown system in the body.

Over time, those with adrenal fatigue end up with depleted and weakened immune systems, finding it difficult to recover from colds, acquiring viral infections that are hard to get over (e.g., mono), or even ending up with a "diagnosis of exclusion": fibromyalgia, chronic fatigue syndrome, etc. Those with true adrenal fatigue will end up with lowered cortisol, and thus less inflammation regulation in the body. In order to improve the anti-inflammatory effects of cortisone and cortisol, the adrenal glands will need to be healed. If you have an autoimmune condition, you will definitely want to make sure your adrenal gland system is being treated, as well as your digestive system and immune system.

Mental Fog and Brain Fatigue

Brain fog, mental fatigue, and inability to focus are common symptoms of an undernourished cellular and mitochondrial system, weakened nervous system, and heightened stress response. Over time, the acute effects of cortisol, which includes improving your ability to focus and helping with retention of short-term memory, flatlines and your brain becomes overwhelmed with the amount of cortisol and neurotransmitters bombarding it, day in and day out.

Your Brain on Stress

It has long been known that conditions such as post-traumatic stress disorder (PTSD) can cause changes in brain configuration by changing the amount of white matter in comparison to gray matter, as well as the size and connectivity of the amygdala, an area of the brain regulating memory, decision-making, and emotional reactions. Gray matter is composed of neurons (bodies of nerve cells); this part of your central nervous system is involved in many of the higher functions, including thinking, reasoning, and decision-making.

The other half of your brain is white matter, which is composed mainly of axons (the tail of the neuron) that connect the neuron bodies to each other and to various regions of the brain. This allows communication to occur between regions of the brain. White matter gets its name because of the fatty myelin sheath that surrounds the axons and allows for a very fast electrical signal to occur, so fast you don't even know it happens.

In a study published in the *Journal of Molecular Psychiatry* in February 2014, researchers found that white matter in animals under stressful situations was being made in excess and was becoming "hardened." This negatively impacted the transmission of signals (communication) because the myelin sheath was getting too large in diameter for appropriate signaling. Normally the brain likes to get rid of extra myelin by "pruning" the fat to maintain the efficiency of transmission of the electrical impulses. This also allows for plasticity in the creation of new pathways in the brain. However, under the recurrent stress, the white matter became more prolific and the gray matter decreased. Thick white matter is a problem because the efficiency of the electrical impulses decreases and nonpruned white matter has more ability to harden, which completely disrupts the signal from making its way to where it needs to.

By focusing on neural stem cell development, the researchers were able to see that those cells under constant influence by cortisol due to post-traumatic stress disorder (PTSD) became oligodendrocytes, which contribute to the myelin sheath and white matter, as opposed to astrocytes, the cells contributing to the gray matter. Thus, over time, more tails were made than bodies. That is a huge problem. Here, you have less efficient transmission of electrical impulses for the brain to communicate and you have shrinking of the gray matter, which means a less dependable higher-functioning center (the neurons send out the communication).

Now, you may not have incurred PTSD, but chronic stress and elevated cortisol, the same mechanisms largely responsible for PTSD, will still have negative repercussions on the same area of your brain over time. What the researchers proposed is that cortisol may be a primary contributor to the hardwiring of the pathways between the hippocampus (area responsible for memory) and the amygdala (responsible for helping with time and place), creating a brain that is predisposed to be in a constant state of fight-or-flight response, creating more states of fear and anxiety, a declining long-term memory, and a disruption in thinking and reasoning.

Fortunately, regular physical activity and mindfulness-based practices are two of the most effective ways to reduce stress, lower cortisol, and protect your brain as it ages. Remember, your brain has a plasticity to it, which means that there is still time. You can change your behaviors and activity to promote a better gray-to-white-matter ratio and to move your body out of constant fight-or-flight readiness. Mindset and behavior are adaptable traits. When you have the right information to change your habits, you can improve your wellness on a daily basis.

FACT

Your brain is super sensitive to the effects of cortisol. When stimulating your brain in the short term, cortisol will help with memory and focus. However, chronic or exaggerated stimulation of the brain by cortisol causes issues with long-term memory, focus, and attention to detail. Be sure to take regular breaks when working on projects. A good rule is 45 minutes of work to a 10-minute break. During that 10 minutes do a physical activity that does not require thought: walking, dishes, vacuuming, raking, etc. This will give your brain the much-needed break it requires to relax from cortisol stimulation.

Inability to Focus and Mental Clarity

Cortisol helps you focus. So why, over time, do you find it hard to do the one thing that cortisol is supposed to make your brain do better? In the short term, cortisol improves your ability to focus on the task at hand and sharpens your short-term memory. However, it is more common to see focus and memory become hazy under the influence of chronic stress. This is probably due to the negative effects cortisol has on the neurons, because of increased oxidative stress and inflammation in the brain as the body tries to keep up with the demand of making stress hormones, and as a result of poor dietary habits, excess caffeine, low intake of antioxidants, and poor detoxification pathways.

CHAPTER 6

Obtaining an Accurate Diagnosis

An estimated four out of five people suffer from adrenal fatigue at some point in their lives. This can include individuals struggling with symptoms from an elevated stress response and high cortisol, and those who are already on their way to adrenal fatigue and cortisol burnout. Knowing where to turn to get an accurate diagnosis is an important step in your journey to heal your adrenal glands. There are signs and symptoms specific to a heightened stress response, as well as signs and symptoms attributable to a poorly functioning hypothalamus-pituitary-adrenal gland (HPA) axis. It is good to be aware of the signs and symptoms that go with both of these, as you may experience some symptoms from your stress response or from a weakened adrenal system—or, more commonly, both. In addition, accurate testing of your adrenal gland hormones will help you understand where you fall on the spectrum of adrenal fatigue.

Adrenal Gland Assessment Questionnaire

You can use the following questionnaire to roughly assess your adrenal gland function based on your signs and symptoms. This is a great foundation for accurately assessing your adrenal gland health. Beyond this assessment, you should get accurate lab testing done to see what your adrenal hormones are telling you about your current physiological state of health.

Adrenal Questionnaire Overview

Answer the following questions about your current state. You can also make note of any past or present symptoms that stand out. The past information will not be used for calculations, but will help give you more information about your level of adrenal gland function, as some individuals have never been well and others experience a gradual decline in adrenal gland function over time. The questionnaire will allow you to fill in whether you experience the symptom mildly, moderately, or severely for your current state. Using the following format, check 1 for mild (rarely or less than monthly), 2 for moderate (weekly or a few times a month), or 3 for severe (experience daily or at least 3–4 times a week). If you don't experience it at all, leave blank.

Your Current Mental and Emotional State

ARE OVERWHELMED EASILY BY STRESS AND PRESSURE*

- 1 _____
- 2 _____
- 3 _____

ARE EASILY OVERWHELMED WITH EMOTION*

- 1 _____
- 2 _____
- 3 _____

APPEAR DRIVEN TO OTHERS, BUT FEEL EXHAUSTED INSIDE*

- 1 _____
- 2 _____
- 3 _____

FEEL EXPLOSIVE OR EXPERIENCE PENT-UP EMOTIONS*

- 1 _____
- 2 _____
- 3 _____

GET WOUND UP EASILY AND FIND IT DIFFICULT TO CALM DOWN*

- 1 _____
- 2 _____
- 3 _____

CONTINUALLY CHECK TO MAKE SURE THINGS ARE DONE, SUCH AS SHUTTING STOVE OFF*

- 1 _____
- 2 _____
- 3 _____

WORRY A LOT ABOUT TERRIBLE THINGS HAPPENING*

- 1 _____
- 2 _____
- 3 _____

WORRY ABOUT EVERYTHING, PLAY BACK SITUATIONS IN YOUR HEAD*

- 1 _____
- 2 _____
- 3 _____

FEEL RESTLESS, DRIVEN, ANXIOUS, AND/OR ON-GUARD*

- 1 _____
- 2 _____
- 3 _____

STAY UP AT NIGHT THINKING ABOUT THE DAY'S EVENTS OR TOMORROW'S TO-DO LIST*

- 1 _____
- 2 _____
- 3 _____

AVOID EMOTIONAL SITUATIONS OR CONFLICT

- 1 _____
- 2 _____
- 3 _____

**HAVE ISSUES WITH FOCUS, SHORT-TERM MEM-
ORY, OR BEING ABLE TO THINK CLEARLY**

- 1 _____
- 2 _____
- 3 _____

**EXPERIENCE FEELINGS OF HOPELESSNESS
OR DESPAIR**

- 1 _____
- 2 _____
- 3 _____

ARE DISTANT WITH OTHERS

- 1 _____
- 2 _____
- 3 _____

EXPERIENCE NERVOUS BREAKDOWNS

- 1 _____
- 2 _____
- 3 _____

MUST FORCE YOURSELF TO KEEP GOING

- 1 _____
- 2 _____
- 3 _____

**HAVE DIFFICULTY ORGANIZING
THOUGHTS**

- 1 _____
- 2 _____
- 3 _____

**HAVE A HARD TIME TRUSTING YOURSELF
TO MAKE DECISIONS**

- 1 _____
- 2 _____
- 3 _____

**FEEL RESTLESS OR ANXIOUS, WHILE ALSO
EXHAUSTED**

- 1 _____
- 2 _____
- 3 _____

ARE FORGETFUL

- 1 _____
- 2 _____
- 3 _____

ARE DEPRESSED OR APATHETIC

- 1 _____
- 2 _____
- 3 _____

Your Current Physical Symptoms

FORGET TO EAT AND DON'T NOTICE, OR FEEL LITTLE APPETITE*
- 1 _____
- 2 _____
- 3 _____

WHEN HUNGRY, GET CONFUSED, SHAKY, IRRITABLE*
- 1 _____
- 2 _____
- 3 _____

SUFFER FROM NERVOUS STOMACH OR INDIGESTION*
- 1 _____
- 2 _____
- 3 _____

HAVE ALLERGIES TO MULTIPLE THINGS, INCLUDING SEASONAL ALLERGIES, PETS, MOLDS*
- 1 _____
- 2 _____
- 3 _____

RUN HOT, OR EXPERIENCE HOT FLASHES, ESPECIALLY AT NIGHT WHILE SLEEPING*
- 1 _____
- 2 _____
- 3 _____

HAVE SKIN ISSUES, INCLUDING THINNING, HIVES, ITCHING FOR NO APPARENT REASON*
- 1 _____
- 2 _____
- 3 _____

EXPERIENCE HEART PALPITATIONS OR POUNDING IN CHEST*
- 1 _____
- 2 _____
- 3 _____

SUFFER FROM ASTHMA OR SEASONAL ALLERGIES*
- 1 _____
- 2 _____
- 3 _____

GET COLD SORES OR CANKER SORES*
- 1 _____
- 2 _____
- 3 _____

ARE EASILY CONSTIPATED OR HAVE INFREQUENT BOWEL MOVEMENTS*
- 1 _____
- 2 _____
- 3 _____

STRUGGLE WITH HIGH BLOOD PRESSURE, HIGH TRIGLYCERIDES, OR DYSLIPIDEMIA (POORLY BALANCED CHOLESTEROL LEVELS)*

- 1 _____
- 2 _____
- 3 _____

EXPERIENCE MUSCLE SPASMS OR CRAMPING*

- 1 _____
- 2 _____
- 3 _____

ARE EASILY SHORT OF BREATH*

- 1 _____
- 2 _____
- 3 _____

SEE, HEAR, OR SMELL THINGS THAT OTHERS DON'T*

- 1 _____
- 2 _____
- 3 _____

GET DIZZY WHEN STANDING UP FROM A SEATED POSITION

- 1 _____
- 2 _____
- 3 _____

NEED TO REST DURING THE DAY, INCLUDING TAKING NAPS

- 1 _____
- 2 _____
- 3 _____

HAVE LOW OR NONEXISTENT SEX DRIVE

- 1 _____
- 2 _____
- 3 _____

HAVE DIFFICULTY LOSING WEIGHT; FEEL PUFFY, POTENTIALLY RETAINING FLUIDS

- 1 _____
- 2 _____
- 3 _____

HAVE DECREASED TOLERANCE FOR COLD, ARE EASILY CHILLED, FEEL COLD WHEN OTHERS APPEAR WARM

- 1 _____
- 2 _____
- 3 _____

GET COLDS OR COUGHS FOR SEVERAL WEEKS TO MONTHS (LONGER THAN OTHERS)

- 1 _____
- 2 _____
- 3 _____

HAVE RHEUMATOID ARTHRITIS OR ANOTHER AUTOIMMUNE CONDITION

- 1 _____
- 2 _____
- 3 _____

HAVE NO ENERGY AND FEEL PHYSICALLY WEAK

- 1 _____
- 2 _____
- 3 _____

EXPERIENCE FATIGUE AFTER EXERTION, RATHER THAN ENERGY

- 1 _____
- 2 _____
- 3 _____

HAVE MULTIPLE SYMPTOMS SUCH AS DIGESTIVE ISSUES, MUSCULOSKELETAL COMPLAINTS, SKIN PROBLEMS, MENTAL/EMOTIONAL IMBALANCES, ETC.

- 1 _____
- 2 _____
- 3 _____

HAVE WORSENING ALLERGIES: MORE SEVERE, MORE FREQUENT, MORE DIVERSE

- 1 _____
- 2 _____
- 3 _____

SUFFER FROM PREMENSTRUAL SYNDROME (PMS)

- 1 _____
- 2 _____
- 3 _____

SWEAT SPONTANEOUSLY DURING THE DAY, BUT GENERALLY RUN COLD

- 1 _____
- 2 _____
- 3 _____

Adrenal Gland Response

EASILY FATIGUED
- 1 _____
- 2 _____
- 3 _____

DIFFICULTY GETTING UP IN THE MORN-ING, EVEN WITH ADEQUATE SLEEP
- 1 _____
- 2 _____
- 3 _____

TIREDNESS IN THE AFTERNOON, OFTEN BETWEEN 2–5 P.M.
- 1 _____
- 2 _____
- 3 _____

ENERGY BURSTS AFTER DINNER
- 1 _____
- 2 _____
- 3 _____

DIFFICULTY FALLING ASLEEP
- 1 _____
- 2 _____
- 3 _____

DIFFICULTY STAYING ASLEEP
- 1 _____
- 2 _____
- 3 _____

SLEEP AIDS OR ALCOHOL REQUIRED IN ORDER TO SLEEP
- 1 _____
- 2 _____
- 3 _____

SWELLING UNDER EYES AFTER RISING THAT GENERALLY GOES AWAY WITHIN A FEW HOURS
- 1 _____
- 2 _____
- 3 _____

BODY PAINFUL TO THE TOUCH
- 1 _____
- 2 _____
- 3 _____

CONSTANT STRESS IN LIFE
- 1 _____
- 2 _____
- 3 _____

MEDICATIONS NEEDED TO MANAGE PAIN (E.G., NSAIDS)
- 1 _____
- 2 _____
- 3 _____

LACK OF ENJOYMENT IN LIFE
- 1 _____
- 2 _____
- 3 _____

LITTLE CONTROL OVER HOW TIME IS SPENT
- 1 _____
- 2 _____
- 3 _____

HEADACHES
- 1 _____
- 2 _____
- 3 _____

Diet and Lifestyle Habits

RELY ON COFFEE OR OTHER STIMULANTS TO GET GOING IN THE MORNING
- 1 _____
- 2 _____
- 3 _____

CRAVE FOODS THAT ARE SALTY
- 1 _____
- 2 _____
- 3 _____

CRAVE FOODS THAT ARE SWEET
- 1 _____
- 2 _____
- 3 _____

CRAVE HIGH-PROTEIN FOODS
- 1 _____
- 2 _____
- 3 _____

FEEL WORSE IF A MEAL IS SKIPPED
- 1 _____
- 2 _____
- 3 _____

USE CAFFEINE LATER IN THE DAY TO STAY AWAKE
- 1 _____
- 2 _____
- 3 _____

USE SUGAR LATER IN THE DAY TO STAY AWAKE
- 1 _____
- 2 _____
- 3 _____

ACTIVELY TRY TO RESTRICT SALT INTAKE
- 1 _____
- 2 _____
- 3 _____

MAKE DIET/FOOD CHOICES THAT ARE UNHEALTHY, SPORADIC, AND UNPLANNED
- 1 _____
- 2 _____
- 3 _____

REQUIRE ONGOING MEALS OR SNACKS TO FEEL BETTER
- 1 _____
- 2 _____
- 3 _____

DO NOT EXERCISE, OR EXERCISE LESS THAN 1–2 TIMES PER WEEK
- 1 _____
- 2 _____
- 3 _____

REQUIRE LYING DOWN DURING THE DAY TO FEEL BETTER
- 1 _____
- 2 _____
- 3 _____

CRAVE A LOT OF FRUIT
- 1 _____
- 2 _____
- 3 _____

Predisposing Factors

ENCOUNTERED LONG PERIODS OF STRESS THAT HAVE AFFECTED HEALTH OR WELLNESS
- 1 _____
- 2 _____
- 3 _____

HAD ONE OR MORE MAJOR STRESSFUL EVENTS IN LIFE (E.G., DEATH OF A LOVED ONE, AUTOMOBILE ACCIDENT)
- 1 _____
- 2 _____
- 3 _____

DRIVEN YOURSELF TO EXHAUSTION
- 1 _____
- 2 _____
- 3 _____

WORKED REALLY HARD WITHOUT PLAY OR RELAXATION IN BETWEEN
- 1 _____
- 2 _____
- 3 _____

GET RECURRENT UPPER RESPIRATORY TRACT INFECTIONS
- 1 _____
- 2 _____
- 3 _____

GET MORE THAN 1–2 COLDS PER YEAR
- 1 _____
- 2 _____
- 3 _____

EASILY GAIN WEIGHT, ESPECIALLY AROUND THE ABDOMEN
- 1 _____
- 2 _____
- 3 _____

HAVE A HISTORY OF ALCOHOL AND/OR DRUG ABUSE
- 1 _____
- 2 _____
- 3 _____

HAVE ENVIRONMENTAL SENSITIVITIES OR ALLERGIES
- 1 _____
- 2 _____
- 3 _____

SUFFER FROM POST-TRAUMATIC STRESS DISORDER
- 1 _____
- 2 _____
- 3 _____

SUFFER FROM ANOREXIA, BULIMIA, OR OTHER EATING DISORDERS
- 1 _____
- 2 _____
- 3 _____

HAVE ONE OR MORE CHRONIC HEALTH CONDITIONS, ILLNESSES, OR DISEASES
- 1 _____
- 2 _____
- 3 _____

HAVE DIABETES, PRE-DIABETES, POLY-CYSTIC OVARY SYNDROME, OR BLOOD SUGAR ISSUES
- 1 _____
- 2 _____
- 3 _____

To tally and evaluate, you will add up all the mild, moderate, and severe responses separately. Take out a piece of paper and make three columns; label them 1: mild, 2: moderate, and 3: severe. Now, go back and count the total number you get for each number. It is easiest to just run through the questionnaire three times; add up all the 1s, then all the 2s, then all the 3s. Do not worry about the asterisk (*) questions right now. This initial tally will help you hone in on the severity of your experiences with adrenal gland dysfunction.

With a higher degree in mild, you are less likely to suffer from adrenal fatigue. You probably just have some level of adrenal "un"-wellness that can be supported with better dietary choices, lifestyle strategies, and minimal therapies to fill up your adrenal bank account. If most of your answers are in the moderate or severe column, then adrenal fatigue is a likely contributor to your symptoms/disease state.

The next step is to get a bird's-eye view on whether you are more in overdrive or under function in your adrenal gland system. Look at the first two sections: "Your Current Mental and Emotional State" and "Your Current Physical Symptoms." Within these sections, you will see asterisks next to the first half of the questions. The asterisk is attached to the questions that are symptoms of hyperadrenia, or over-simulation from the adrenal system. The questions without an asterisk point to hypoadrenia, or adrenal fatigue/burnout. Use that same piece of paper and make two columns: Label the first column *, and label the second column no*.

Count up the total number of symptoms you marked with an asterisk, from both sections (no need to separate sections), versus the total number without an asterisk. It does not matter whether the mark is mild, moderate, or severe. If you have more checks with an asterisk, it is an indicator that you may be in adrenal overdrive.

This questionnaire is just an initial tool, however. To really know if you are in hyperadrenia or hypoadrenia, appropriate lab work is encouraged. Lab work tells you when your cortisol is high or low at four specific times throughout the day, and this will allow you to get specific with your treatment plan.

Getting More Specific with Diagnosis

For the most accurate analysis, getting laboratory testing is the next best step. It is important to have a qualified practitioner look at your symptoms objectively, and put together your current state of health with a comprehensive intake, which includes a well taken medical history, a review of your current symptoms, a review of the function of your systems, an understanding of your lifestyle and dietary habits, and your social, emotional, spiritual, and psychological behaviors. This will provide you with about 80 percent of the information needed to understand how best to treat and heal the root cause of your adrenal fatigue. The adrenal fatigue questionnaire is a great starting place, and can alert you to whether your adrenal glands are likely over- or underfunctioning. The adrenal gland testing will help you hone in on an individualized treatment for yourself.

Why Conventional Medicine Misses the Diagnosis

Since the symptoms of adrenal fatigue are so varied, it is extremely difficult for practitioners of conventional medicine to wrap their heads around it as a diagnosis. And even if they did, would they know what to do with the information? Modern medicine tends to compartmentalize the body, as if it were a piece of machinery with independently functioning parts. But the body is not a piece of machinery; each of its systems interacts with every other system. So if you have a problem in one system, there is a high likelihood that another system upstream or downstream from the one experiencing symptoms will also be weakened or compromised.

Another reason current medical practice isn't adept at treating chronic disease and adrenal gland function is because the focus is on managing symptoms, or on the flip side, trying to make them disappear. When the medication is removed, the symptom will still be there. Therefore, the disease process is still occurring whether the symptom is "wellcontrolled" or not.

Combining those two weaknesses opens up a whole slew of problems for actually healing the body and maintaining health. For instance, high blood pressure is inherently harsh on the capillaries and the kidneys, as well as other areas in the body such as the brain, the heart itself, etc. By just lowering blood pressure, there is a slight reduction in the amount of pressure on the heart and the vasculature, but that reduction is only maintained while the medication is being used. Blood pressure is often managed with multiple medications and with regular increases in medications because the underlying issue has never been addressed.

ALERT

In the United States, about 77.9 million (1 out of every 3) adults have high blood pressure. Because medications alone only control blood pressure, rather than heal it, it is best to make sure that you include the following therapies to help your body work to lower blood pressure naturally: lose excess weight, increase potassium intake and magnesium intake, restrict caffeine and alcohol, increase fiber, increase consumption of fruits and vegetables, and increase physical activity or exercise.

When you have symptoms in various parts of your body, as you do with adrenal fatigue, it is common to have treatments for each individual symptom. It is not common for the medical system to put all the symptoms together. The current paradigm of treating symptoms with drugs, in a very disjointed manner, where one specialist may not know what you have been prescribed by another specialist, where insurance companies tell doctors what they can and cannot diagnose and bill, where synthetic drugs are the mainstay of treatment, and where the body is not looked at as a holistic being, needing support for physical, spiritual, mental, and emotional ailments, is slowly transforming.

What Testing to Avoid

It is not appropriate to just get one blood cortisol reading to evaluate your adrenal glands. Your adrenal system works in a circadian rhythm; therefore, taking only one "picture" of the adrenal system via blood cortisol gives you absolutely no information on how the release of cortisol is working over the 24-hour period. As mentioned in previous chapters, the circadian rhythm, otherwise known as the sleep-wake cycle, is the natural rhythm that your body goes through over 24 hours. During the circadian rhythm, you are awake and energized and releasing lots of cortisol, or asleep, repairing, restoring, and releasing less cortisol. In order to appropriately evaluate how your adrenal glands are functioning, you need to get multiple readings of your cortisol over a day.

Other tests that may not be great at helping you understand your adrenal health in its natural circadian rhythm include the 24-hour urine test, which can be used to evaluate your total cortisol over a 24-hour period. This test gives you the results of your total cortisol output, so treatment is not specific enough to correct for when cortisol is low and when it is elevated. In addition, doing challenge tests, such as the ACTH (adrenocorticotropic hormone) test, is not appropriate for the vast majority of adrenal fatigue sufferers, because you are most likely not a candidate for being diagnosed with Addison's or pituitary gland insufficiency. Lastly, the single blood draw "snapshot" of cortisol is not helpful at all either, because it does not depict the natural cortisol rhythm over an entire day.

Adrenal Testing Overview

In order to properly assess the health of your adrenal glands, you should take four readings of your cortisol level over the course of one day. Doing so is necessary because of the sleep-wake cycle and the general nature of cortisol. Cortisol is released throughout the day in a rhythmic manner. Therefore, having an understanding of what fluctuations are occurring in your cortisol and adrenal hormone output is the best way to begin to treat the adrenal glands holistically.

Cortisol Lab Test

The best test to get to examine your cortisol levels is a salivary test. These tests are minimally invasive, and only require several spit collections through the course of a day. They are relatively inexpensive compared with other laboratory tests, and they are easily collected in your house (rather than a lab), so they can be used to monitor treatment.

The most important reason to use these tests, though, is that the salivary labs measure "free" hormones, ones that are readily being used by the cells. Hormones in your body can be either bound to a protein and carried around the bloodstream or unconnected to a protein, free and able to activate target tissues. The ones that we are most interested in are the free hormones. Because the saliva serves as a filter for blood, the proteins don't easily get through, so most of the hormones in the saliva are free. This varies with different hormones, but free cortisol moves easily into the saliva from the blood, and thus is a good candidate for salivary testing.

You will want to collect at least four samples over the course of the day. The ideal times to collect samples are 6–7 A.M., 11 A.M.–12 P.M., 4–6 P.M., and 10 P.M.–12 A.M. Of course, adjusting the "clock" to your symptoms is advisable as well. If insomnia is one of your main complaints, then you can do your late-night collection between 12 A.M.–1 A.M. The afternoon collection can be closer to 4 P.M. than 6 P.M., if that is when you feel your worst energy slump. The main point is to do at least four saliva tests over the course of one day.

DHEA Lab Test

Another test you should get is DHEA-S (dehydroepiandrosterone-sulfate), because the adrenal glands are the primary source of this hormone. DHEA-S is the active form of DHEA, and is a reflection of the health of the area in the adrenal glands responsible for the sex hormones. DHEA is a precursor to mainly androgens (e.g., testosterone) and estrogen. DHEA-S is often low in adrenal fatigue, and in cases where cortisol elevation is prominent.

The average amount of DHEA made daily is 25mg, and this decreases as you age. DHEA is often sold as the "anti-aging hormone," but you will need a lot more than just DHEA to age gracefully. When DHEA levels are low, you don't have enough precursor hormone to make your sex hormones. This deficiency will increase feelings of malaise, lack of interest in life, and general unwellness. Very often other symptoms of a hormonal imbalance will be experienced.

Additional Lab Tests for Adrenal Function

Melatonin is another hormone to consider getting tested, especially if your sleep cycle is disrupted. Often this is a urine test, and you can compare your melatonin output at various times of the day in conjunction with cortisol output.

Secretory immunoglobulin A (SIgA), sometimes also called salivary IgA, lab testing may be considered, especially if any of the following symptoms are present: digestive symptoms, allergies, sensitivities to food or environmental allergens, frequent colds, difficulty recovering from yearly colds. SIgA lives in the mucous membranes and is your first line of defense against microbial invaders including bacteria, yeast, viruses, and parasites. This immunoglobulin is often low in those with adrenal fatigue who also have the previously mentioned symptoms. Knowing this can help you treat the low SIgA in conjunction with the adrenal gland treatment.

Additional Testing Done at Home

There are a few self-tests you can do at home to see if you are a good candidate for an adrenal fatigue diagnosis. Be aware that these tests won't tell you exactly what degree your adrenal fatigue has reached and don't give you a good picture of the circadian rhythm. With that said, being able to take control of your health and have tools to understand where your health stands is always empowering.

Iris Contraction Test

This test looks at the contractibility of the iris. The iris is the circular muscle that contracts and relaxes the pupil. In a healthy individual, the iris should constrict when subjected to light, and then as the iris is continually exposed to the light it should remain constricted. In an individual with hypoadrenia, the pupil is unable to hold the contraction and will dilate despite the light continually being shined on it. Often, the pupil dilation occurs for a longer period of time with more severe cases of adrenal fatigue. This is a fun test to do if you are being treated for adrenal fatigue, and can be done on a monthly basis to see how you're responding to treatment. To accurately document this, you'll want to time how many seconds, within a 2-minute window, the pupil remains dilated with a flashlight shining in your eye in a dark room after the initial contraction, and keep track of that as you continue your treatment.

Postural Hypotension

This test measures blood pressure. One of the most common reasons for low blood pressure is low adrenal gland function. If your blood pressure drops upon standing up from lying down, this often indicates hypoadrenia. To do this at home, all you need is a blood pressure cuff that can also measure your heart rate. You will want to lie down in a quiet place for 10 minutes and then take your blood pressure while still lying down. Next you will stand up and measure your blood pressure upon standing. Normally blood pressure should rise 10–20mmHg, just from standing up. If the blood pressure does not increase or decreases at least 10mmHg, then you have some degree of hypoadrenia. The more it decreases, the worse the diagnosis.

Sergent's White Line

This test assesses the capillary response. The test is a simple test done on the skin of your abdomen. With either your fingernail or the dull end of a piece of silverware, run a line along your stomach. In a healthy individual, the line will turn white immediately and then turn red within a few seconds. In those with hypoadrenia, either the line will remain white for longer than 2–3 seconds or the line will widen. This test is only accurate in about 40 percent of those with moderate to severe hypoadrenia. However, being able to test yourself at home gives you the power to understand your own body!

QUESTION

Why is it important to get the right lab tests to assess your adrenal gland function?
The adrenal hormone cortisol is released in a rhythm over the course of the day. By just measuring one cortisol reading, you will not get a clear picture of what cortisol release looks like over the day. Likewise, if you collect a 24-hour specimen of cortisol without knowing how much you released at specific times throughout the day, you will be left with only a single number. These tests are not helpful for really understanding what the adrenal glands are doing over the course of the day, and more importantly, without knowing what cortisol release looks like, treatment cannot get as specific as you need.

Additional Testing Beyond Adrenals

Depending on your signs and symptoms, you may consider additional testing beyond the normal adrenal stress testing. For instance, if some of your symptoms are hormonal, you would consider testing hormones such as the various estrogens, progesterone, testosterone, and their metabolites (a breakdown product of metabolism). If some of your symptoms are mental or emotional, including having difficulty focusing or experiencing brain fog/fatigue, you may consider looking at a complete neurotransmitter lab to evaluate for an imbalance in this area. If you also have symptoms of the digestive system, you would want targeted laboratory tests to rule out conditions such as yeast, mold, or nonbeneficial bacterial overgrowth, small intestinal bacterial overgrowth (SIBO), or food sensitivities. Again, if you have a complex medical history or are experiencing multiple symptoms in various systems, working with a professional is the best way to have an objective treatment and accurate guidance on how to heal your symptoms and transition to a preventative lifestyle.

Putting the Pieces Together: You Are Unique

Most individuals with any sort of adrenal fatigue symptoms will be considered "healthy." When having your adrenal gland laboratory testing done, it is important to understand that labs have a mean average built into them, based on these "healthy" populations. Labs are one piece of the pie. It is necessary for you to take all of your signs and symptoms, past medical history, and standard laboratory blood tests as well as the adrenal gland testing and put them all together to get the most accurate diagnosis.

Some individuals may have cortisol in the afternoon that is "normal," but this is the part of the day that is the most difficult as far as symptoms are concerned. You can see this commonly on blood tests, where there is a "normal" range of lab values. However, what if your lab value is in the low normal range or the high normal range? Are you still normal? Oftentimes, no. The most common lab this happens with is thyroid testing, where an individual will still be within the normal range although the TSH is approaching hypothyroidism. Nothing will be done for the individual until the lab value is abnormal. The focus is on symptom management only, not the prevention of disease, so you only get a diagnosis of disease when there is complete abnormality.

The best way to help yourself and get specific information about healing symptoms is to put together the pieces of your unique puzzle. This includes your current signs and symptoms, medical history, family history, dietary and lifestyle habits, and pertinent lab testing. Don't wait until labs are completely abnormal before doing something. The best medicine is preventative medicine, and once your adrenal glands are healing, you're on the right road to keeping yourself healthy into old age.

CHAPTER 7

Healing Adrenal Fatigue: Starting with the Basics

Your diet is the most important and crucial part of your wellness plan. What you put in your mouth matters to your health. One of the worst things you can do is fall into the trap of "going on a diet." Instead, you need to think about diet as what you eat, day in and day out. This is how you will succeed with your diet. What you should do is make adjustments in your diet to create a healthful relationship with food. You, like many people, may struggle with food addictions, cravings, and intense emotional feelings in connection with food. The more you stay off the self-defeating path and get rid of the foods that keep you in that unhealthy cycle, the better off you and your vital health will be.

Let's Start Here When It Comes to Healing Adrenal Glands

Healing the HPA axis can take some thoughtful investigation depending on where you are on the road of hypoadrenia. If you have MSS1, your treatment will be different from MSS2, and so forth. Your treatment will also vary depending on what other symptoms you have.

However, there are commonalities to treating all stages of adrenal fatigue. Once you identify your symptoms, you can add on the specific dietary recommendations for your stage of adrenal fatigue. From there you should add on specific lifestyle therapies to help you recover from adrenal fatigue by balancing your stress response in your daily life. Lastly, you can use all the various natural therapy recommendations to improve upon diet, lifestyle, and stress management techniques to give yourself the most rounded healing plan.

FACT

Your adrenal glands will only heal when you give them all the right conditions and environment to do so. This means your treatment plan should address the physical, mental, and emotional aspects of who you are. You will also need to make sure your diet and lifestyle, as well as the natural supplements you use, are all specific to your stage of adrenal fatigue. The natural therapies do wonders, but they are nothing without the foundation of your diet and lifestyle habits.

Change Your Response to Stress

This is the most crucial piece of advice for healing the adrenal glands and keeping them healthy. The way you manage your stress—e.g., by internalizing it and allowing it to affect your body—is a major reason why you may have adrenal fatigue. Correcting this, along with allowing appropriate recovery times and support between stressful events, will carry a lot of the healing journey for you. This is not necessarily an easy practice, but at the end of the day, you will get a lot further the more you can transform your response to stress.

Remember, stress is not going anywhere, nor would you want it to, as it does serve as a perfect survival mechanism. You just don't want it to be the reason you don't feel like yourself. All the daily lifestyle habits you learn to use will help you change your response to stress, as will developing the mindset to do it. Rather than thinking about how to get rid of stress, you should begin to think about how you can react differently to a stressful situation next time. For instance, rather than dreading whatever brings you the most stress in the day, you can learn to make peace with it.

Remove Toxicity from Your Life

What exactly are toxic things? This could be people, relationships, activities, skin care and cleaning products, your dietary choices, and so much more. It is so taxing and draining having a relationship with someone who just takes and doesn't give. These people may ask you to do a lot for them without much gratitude, expect you to move the world for them, fill your head with rumors, gossips, and lies. Your intuition tells you to stay away, but you have yet to "cut the cord" on this relationship.

You already know that your adrenal glands respond to your physiology and biochemistry. When you are under attack emotionally, whether directly by being put down or indirectly by lowering your vibration and being part of gossip or lies, your body is under stress. And the longer you take the assaults, the longer the stress response remains elevated. Next time, politely excuse yourself or let this person know you have needs and feelings too.

Increase the Deposits Made to the Adrenal Bank Account

Increasing the deposits made into your adrenal bank account is a huge part of healing your adrenal glands and promoting long-term health. The way you feel today is the culmination of everything you have done up until now. Your life is made up of daily activities and habits that you do either because you have to, you want to, or you just do without really knowing why. And everything you do affects your health and ultimately your quality of life. You have the ability to flip your disease-promoting habits into health-promoting habits.

ESSENTIAL

Adrenal deposits include: drinking adequate amounts of water, eating a balanced meal, removing sugar from your diet, spending time outdoors in the fresh air, exercising, getting 8 hours of sleep, and so on. You want to try to avoid unnecessary withdrawals, so there will be plenty of deposits still available when stressors come along and start making withdrawals. Withdrawals include: caffeine, soda, a sedentary lifestyle, processed foods, sugar, living on autopilot, feeling rushed or late all the time, and so forth.

Clean Up Your Diet

If your diet is filled with microwave meals, "food-like" products, and foods that have an ingredient list with words you don't even know how to pronounce, you are going to feel lacking in energy and vitality. Think about it: When you buy an apple, it is full of nutrition that slowly degrades over time. It, like you, is alive. If you feed your body "apple-flavored" doughnuts, you should expect absolutely no nutritional value from that food, especially if it expires in 6, 12, 18 months. Food, unless it is naturally canned and preserved, is not meant to last, because it, like you, is a living organism. You get the nutrition that runs all your biochemical pathways from living food.

Your (Healthy) Diet

Your diet is at the heart of your medicine. As Hippocrates said, "Let food be thy medicine and medicine be thy food." Think of food like the fuel in your car. You know that your car uses gas in order to run, so are you going to put water in it? Paint? Other liquid? No! You are going to put fuel in it.

Your body needs food to run—whole foods, which provide you with all the healthy fats, complex carbohydrates, proteins, and phytochemicals (hundreds of nutrients, vitamins, and minerals). Your body does not do well on food-like substances.

The Grocery Store Rule

If you were to walk into a grocery store and remain only in the perimeter of the store, plus the bulk aisle, you would find all the whole foods your body needs to stay nourished. You start in produce, and then move to the fish and meat, dairy, deli, and so on. You take a stroll down the aisle where you can get healthy oils, whole beans and grains, raw nuts and seeds, and maybe a few odds and ends such as coconut oil or tamari. For the most part, your diet should only consist of these foods or ones located in the areas mentioned.

Why is this diet vital to adrenal health? Well, it's not. It is actually vital to whole health! If you want to heal your adrenal glands and your body, you need to be providing them with nutrients to fuel biochemical pathways daily. Every day of your life you have the opportunity to lay the foundation of good health, and that starts with what you eat. This approach to eating will provide you with energy, vitality, improved sleep quality, and so much more.

Diet Dos and Don'ts

The health world is pretty much riddled with a million hypotheses on what is healthy and what is not. For you to be able to navigate these theories, you need to know which ones to rely on. These tenets will be like your North Star when it comes to diet. If you follow them, you will not be led astray when evaluating if something is good for you or not.

Eat Whole Foods

If you predominantly eat whole foods—apples, asparagus, quinoa, wild-caught salmon, etc.—you are well on your way to having a diet that supports your biochemistry, heals your adrenal fatigue, and keeps you healthy long into old age.

If you refer back to the Grocery Store Rule and you find that most of your shopping is done in the aisles, you are not eating mostly whole foods. Even at natural food stores, the aisles are filled with processed foods.

Throw Out the Calories

If a diet makes you count calories, or even worse, makes you keep track of points when it comes to food, there is little use for it. The only counting that is really beneficial is if you are trying to keep track of your carbohydrate-protein-fat ratio, which is slightly different for each person depending on your level of adrenal fatigue and corresponding symptoms. Those with more severe adrenal fatigue need more healthy carbohydrates and protein to keep blood sugar in balance and prevent the breakdown of muscle for glucose (muscle is made of amino acids, similar to protein). Counting your dietary intake of carbohydrate-protein-fat is most helpful when transitioning to a new, healthier way of eating. Counting the intake of other key nutrients from your food can be beneficial too, depending on your symptoms and needs. For instance, the best place to get calcium is from food, and then supplement as needed. So you can fill out a calcium intake to see if you are getting your needs met through diet, and then if you are not, you can supplement more specifically for your dietary gaps.

Eat Fermented Foods

Foods that are fermented or cultured contain a lot of living (and dead) micro-organisms that you would not be alive without. You absolutely need to be giving your body and digestive system foods such as yogurt, kimchee, sauerkraut, kombucha, and kefir on a daily basis. Plan on eating a little bit of cultured or fermented foods with at least one meal daily to start out, and as it becomes more habitual for you to eat these foods, start adding them to various meals throughout the day. The health effects are astounding.

QUESTION

How much water is needed for health?
Your body is 70 percent water and requires adequate water replenishment daily to function normally. Water is needed to keep your blood fluid, balance blood pressure, and support your adrenals. Oftentimes, just drinking adequate amounts of water daily will boost your energy. If you haven't been drinking enough water for your body size, simply start today. As you add more water, you may find you need to go to the bathroom more. This is normal as you move from a dehydrated state to a hydrated one, and will slow down the more you consume the right daily amount for you.

Liquids/Hydration

The best liquid you can drink is filtered water. You really can't get much better than that, except maybe herbal tea, because then you are also giving your body some great medicine. You should shoot for roughly half your body weight in ounces of water a day. So if you weigh 130 pounds, shoot for 65 ounces of water. You may find that with exercise and caffeine consumption you require more. Liquids should not be consumed with a meal, as they dilute digestive juices and make it harder for your stomach and intestines to do the good work they are supposed to. Use minimal liquids to wash meals down, and instead enjoy liquids throughout the day between meals.

Other healthy liquids include: kombucha, raw milk, some alternative milks (e.g., organic almond or hazelnut), organic coffee, and organic green tea. Try to avoid soymilk, juices, sodas, and too many caffeinated beverages. Even 100 percent fruit juice, unless freshly squeezed, has degraded and lost most of its nutrients due to sitting on a shelf. If you juice yourself, it is best to consume fresh-pressed juices within 30 minute of making it. If you are interested in juicing, a masticating juicer is a better way to go, as it leaves much of the fiber in there, making for a more "whole" juice.

Caffeine

Caffeine has a lot of redeeming qualities, but it also is really not the best chemical if you suffer from adrenal fatigue. If you experience cortisol dips and tend to crave a pick-me-up in the middle of the day, you may find yourself turning to coffee. Often those in MSS2, where cortisol output is elevated, will crave coffee and sugars, almost like the body is saying keep this "high" going. However, you are just asking the adrenals to put out even more cortisol. This can inadvertently lead to heart palpitations, anxiety, insomnia, and more. If you need an afternoon pick-me-up, organic green tea would be the best thing to transition to if you rely on coffee. Even better would be herbal tea, and another completely different option would be to get outside for 15 minutes and take a brisk walk. Often, you just have to break the cycle of bad habits, and you can start to make new, good ones.

Organic, Non-GMO, and Local

When it comes to eating whole foods and cleaning up your diet, it is important to eat as naturally as possible, and that includes reducing the likelihood that your food will come with something toxic on it. Remember that pesticides and herbicides are designed to hurt the nervous systems of critters. You can be sure they have an effect on you, too (though not as drastic).

The best place to turn for reliable information is the Environmental Working Group (*www.ewg.org*). Every year, they release their organic shopper's guide, which has the Dirty Dozen Plus and Clean Fifteen lists. These are the fruits and vegetables you either must buy organic (Dirty Dozen Plus) or can get away with buying nonorganic (Clean Fifteen). Everything else sort of falls in the middle, and will depend on your budget.

Non-GMO (genetically modified organism) is an organism that has not been altered by man and then bred to prevent disease or promote crop production. Classically, GMO crops are patented gene splicing. There are many reasons not to put GMOs in your body. While those who support the use of GMOs would like the masses to believe that it is better because crop yields are bigger and not as much pesticides need to be sprayed, you have to remember that as a species, human beings have evolved right next to the foods they currently eat, not with some genetically manipulated corn, soy, or potato. There is increasing evidence in the scientific community that GMO crops are causing health issues.

ALERT

Genetically modified (GM) crops are not the answer to world hunger. A major United Nations and World Bank–sponsored report compiled by 400 scientists and endorsed by 58 countries concluded that GM crops have little to offer global agriculture and the challenges of poverty, hunger, and climate change, because better alternatives are available.

The local food movement has increased food coming from local economies, which means that small farmers are being better supported and you get fresher food because it doesn't need to travel thousands of miles halfway around the world. When it comes to buying local and organic, or local and non-GMO, or local, organic, and non-GMO, you will need to make those decisions yourself.

Cortisol and Blood Sugar Control Through Your Diet

Cortisol is a glucocorticoid; it controls blood sugar levels. *Gluco-* refers to glucose, being blood glucose or blood sugar. When you are in MSS2–MSS3, your blood sugar levels will be up and down. Adhering to a dietary plan that helps you keep your blood sugar in better balance is key. As you move to MSS0–MSS1, or if you are starting out there, your blood sugar is not being as badly imbalanced by cortisol, and you will find it easier to move from burning glucose to burning fat (ketogenesis). The latter is much healthier for long-term health and longevity. When you burn fat, you are continually turning over your fat stores. You are less likely to store toxic chemicals (stored in fat), and your body ages more slowly.

When you are in MSS2, hyperadrenia, your cortisol levels are overall higher and this means that you are breaking down more glycogen (the storage form of glucose) and putting more glucose out into your bloodstream on a regular basis. This stimulates insulin release from the pancreas. However, cortisol likes to interfere with insulin's actions at the receptor sites. You end up with insulin desensitization, a common early finding in type 2 diabetes. If you have MSS2 and a family history of diabetes, there is no better time than the present to heal your adrenal glands.

When you are in MSS3, hypoadrenia, your cortisol is low overall and your body won't have enough blood glucose to fuel its needs. You most likely experience feelings of low blood sugar (hypoglycemia), which are shakiness, light-headedness, irritability, and/or anxiety without food. For both MSS2 and MSS3, eating regularly every 2–3 hours is key. And the meals and snacks should be a nice mixture of complex carbohydrates, protein, and healthy fats.

Snack Ideas

Snack time is very important for you if you are in the MSS2–MSS3 stage of adrenal fatigue. Snacks will keep your blood sugar in better balance and help you heal your adrenals. Providing yourself with food more regularly in these advanced stages of adrenal fatigue is necessary so that the adrenals don't have to work harder than they should. The goal is to have your adrenals rest and repair as much as possible.

Use the snack list at the end of this section to help you prep your snacks each week. You may find that prepping snacks 1–2 times during the week, say on Sunday and Wednesday, makes for less work and a better weekday meal plan. Don't rely on getting food on the go. While you want to stream-line your food production needs (by prepping a few times each week), you definitely don't want to eat convenience foods, such as bagels, chips, and candy, because they are not generally healthy.

One great versatile snack is vegetable sticks. Some ideas include: car-rots, celery, cucumbers, tomatoes, peppers, and radishes. Grabbing a handful of these each day will take care of one snack time. You can essentially pair these with any of your favorite protein choices. For fruit, you should ideally stick to what is local. If you have apples, pears, and berries growing locally, choose to eat those. Tropical fruit is fine as well, but remember that tropical fruits are higher in sugars, so they aren't the best choice for continued blood sugar balancing.

With raw nuts and seeds, choose varieties such as pumpkin, sunflower, walnut, almond, pecan, Brazil, cashew, and hazelnut. Peanuts aren't nuts; they are a legume. You are better off staying away from peanuts and peanut but-ter as they are one of the most common foods contaminated with aflatoxin (toxic metabolite produced by fungi), along with corn and cottonseed oil. Nuts and seeds are dense, so make sure you don't consume any more than ⅓ cup of seeds, and no more than what can fit in your palm for nuts—for instance, about 20–25 almonds is a serving, whereas 3–4 Brazil nuts is a serving.

SNACK LIST
- Cut-up vegetables with almond butter or hummus
- Cut-up vegetables with black bean dip or guacamole
- Cut-up vegetables with yogurt (whole or 2%) or cheese
- Cut-up vegetables with sliced all-natural turkey or chicken
- Fruit with yogurt (whole or 2%) or cheese
- Handful of raw nuts or seeds and a piece of fruit
- Hard-boiled egg(s)
- Apple or celery with almond butter, cashew butter, or sunflower butter

CHAPTER 8

Food Matters,
and So Does Your Digestion

What you eat, when you eat, and how you create your meals are important factors in healing your adrenal fatigue. The following sections will give you some information about what a healthy meal plan looks like for your stage of adrenal fatigue, as well as what you should be including from each basic food group. This won't be the standard American diet pyramid. Instead, these foods focus on adrenal health and whole body health.

The Quality of Your Food Matters

What food you buy, where you buy it, what your food contains, and how you prepare it all matter significantly to your health. Your shopping cart should be filled with the following food categories as 80 percent of your shopping needs. The other 20 percent can be the foods that are more your comfort food. Obviously striving for anything over 80 percent is just going to provide you with that much more benefit to healing your adrenal glands and living a preventative lifestyle.

Vegetables and Fruit

Produce should be bought as fresh as possible, and preferably seasonally. Why not eat some local blueberries or blackberries, or local apples or pears. There is an ever-increasing support for bringing more local food to local markets. This means you not only get what grows near you, but you get food that is much fresher. For the most part, the longer the food can stay on the plant it grows from, the more nutritious it will be.

If you are not familiar with community supported agriculture (CSA) initiatives, please check out the resources listed in Appendix B and get online. Farms are popping up all over, and joining a CSA allows you to get local food in your area as well as support your local farmers. It is a double win.

ALERT

Cans are lined with bisphenol-A (BPA), a plastic that is a known endocrine disruptor. Try to avoid as much commercially canned food as possible, which is different from canning your own food. There are canned products you can find if you enjoy foods such as coconut milk, whose manufacturers don't use BPA. Please note that there may be other plastics used in these cans.

When buying produce at the grocery store, fresh is best, frozen is second, and canned should be avoided. There really is no need for canned vegetables unless you are making yourself a survival kit or want to donate to a food pantry. Canned vegetables are highly lacking in nutrition from being overly processed, and even BPA-free cans are not free of plastics.

When buying vegetables, the best rule is to go for the rainbow. You want vegetables of all colors so you get a nice array of phytonutrients in your diet. Yes, there are vitamins and minerals found in these vegetables, but there are hundreds of other plant chemicals that may be even more protective than just your run-of-the mill vitamins A, B, and C.

ESSENTIAL

Vegetables are crucial for overall health. The majority of your vitamins and minerals come from these wonderful foods and should be a staple with nearly every meal. Some of the healthiest vegetables are the cruciferous veggies including kale, broccoli, cabbage, and cauliflower; green leafy veggies including arugula, mustard, and chard; allium veggies which include onion, garlic, scallions, and leeks; avocados; mushrooms; and the "rainbow" of vegetables including beets, sweet potatoes, summer squash, zucchini, blue potatoes, and eggplant to name a few.

Meat: Beef, Bison, Turkey, Chicken, Duck

Meat can be a great food to have in your diet. Traditionally, our ancestors would eat organ meats with a bit of muscle meat. Today, you most likely eat tons of muscle meat and not much organ meat (if any). Organ meat and muscle meat should be from organic or non-hormone, non-antibiotic sources. You should look into meat shares in your local community, as many farmers are now offering quarter, half, and whole cuts of meat, all butchered. You may even want to look at local CSA farms in your area that are growing vegetables and/or fruit and see which farms may also be offering meat and dairy.

Organ meat, from organic sources, can be really healthy for your body, especially for those in more deficient states such as MSS3. These meats often contain many more nutrients than just the standard protein and fat. For instance, heart muscle contains more CoQ10 than any other piece of meat. Liver *is one* of the best sources of choline and B_{12}. Bone broths are another extremely healthy food from animals. These can be made by utilizing a left-over carcass, as the case with chicken or turkey, or by purchasing bones and other animal parts (e.g., pigs' feet) from your local butcher. These broths are naturally high in nutrients, amino acids, gelatin, and collagen.

Fish and Shellfish

Seafood is a very healthy form of food. Unfortunately, because of ocean pollution, you will need to be careful about what you are buying so you don't inadvertently increase your levels of mercury or expose yourself to too much PCB (polychlorinated biphenyl). You will want to look at the Environmental Working Group's information about chemical levels in seafood, safe fish and shellfish sold for consumption, and recommended monthly consumption to stay below certain levels of these chemicals.

Please note that there are chemicals in land meat as well, so don't think avoiding fish and just consuming land animals will prevent you from being exposed. You just have to be smart about what you buy. You will also want to make sure you consume wild-caught seafood. Farm-raised fish add a huge unsustainable and toxic burden to the ocean, and are generally a lower nutritional–quality food.

Dairy

Dairy can be very healthy for you if you tolerate it well. Cultured dairy is often the best choice, and can be eaten by many people with lactose intolerance. Dairy, just like meat, should come from non-hormone, non-antibiotic sources. Try to stay away from fat-free and instead go for options such as 2% and whole, as the fat in dairy, in moderate amounts, is quite healthy and helps you absorb all the fat-soluble vitamins from the milk.

Cultured foods such as yogurt and kefir are great for the digestive system and the immune system. There are a lot of options for those who cannot tolerate cow's milk, including goat, sheep, buffalo, and ewe. Raw milk is quite healthy, and there are many raw milk producers turning up in states where raw milk is allowed. These facilities are closely monitored and many of them are much cleaner than the generic milk you get at the convenience or chain grocery store.

Grains and Beans

Grains and beans are definitely one of those in-again, out-again foods. If you are going to eat them, soak your grains and beans so that the outer shell is cracked open and chemicals such as phytic acid are neutralized. Grains and beans (and nuts and seeds) contain phytic acid so that animals will leave them alone in the wild.

What is the problem with phytic acid? It reduces the absorption of minerals by binding to these minerals and making them less available to you. What can you do about that if you enjoy rice and beans? By soaking the beans in warm water overnight, you greatly reduce the content of phytic acid and increase your absorption of minerals. But you absolutely should avoid these if you aren't going to do the work to cook them correctly. As for soy, since the topic is beans, if you are going to consume it, it really should only be fermented (e.g., tempeh and miso), as this improves digestibility of the bean, provides you with higher K2 levels from the food, and gives your body lots of probiotics.

Raw Nuts and Seeds

Nuts and seeds are quite healthy, but they have the same issue with phytic acid. These foods contain healthy omega fats, protein, and fat-soluble vitamins, as well as fiber. Nuts and seeds should either be consumed raw or soaked/fermented to improve digestibility and micronutrient values. Roasted nuts and seeds have a more likely chance of being or becoming rancid. You can dry-roast your own soaked nuts and seeds in a dehydrator if you prefer a crunchier nut or seed. As mentioned earlier, it is also advisable to stay away from peanuts, as these are not nuts, but legumes, and technically should be cooked the way other beans are cooked.

Your Meal Plan: What and When to Eat

What you eat is going to be fairly consistent between the different stages of adrenal fatigue, though you may find that your protein needs are higher in the MSS3 stage than in the other stages. Keeping blood sugar in balance with a nice variety of foods in the MSS2–MSS3 stages is key. You will eat whole foods as the base of your diet, meaning that when you buy a food, you are able to say what it is, in a few words: kale, quinoa, Cheddar cheese, chicken thighs, etc. When you buy packaged foods, they should have a relatively short list of ingredients—try to stick to fewer than seven—and the ingredients should all be words you can identify. If you can't pronounce it, best to avoid it, or at the very least look it up to see what it comes from!

Protein, Complex Carbohydrates, and Fats

Protein needs in MSS2–MSS3 will be a little different. Those in MSS2 will likely do well with 1.2gm/kg, which is slightly higher than the 1.0gm/kg recommended for "normal" healthy adults in MSS0–MSS1 (e.g. if you are a bodybuilder you need more). If you are in MSS3, you may find that you need to eat 1.3–1.4gm/kg to keep your energy levels stable over the course of the day. As your adrenals heal, you can eat less protein as your meals can become farther apart, since blood sugar balancing will not be so vital with a healthy adrenal gland system.

Complex carbohydrates come in the form of grains, beans, and vegetables. You should primarily eat them as starchy vegetables: parsnip, beet, plantain, red and purple potato, pumpkin, acorn squash, spaghetti squash, butternut squash, delicata squash, yams, sweet potatoes, green peas, cassava, zucchini, and yellow squash. Healthy grains include: quinoa, millet, amaranth, rice, oats, buckwheat, and barley. Oats are often processed in a facility that contains wheat, so if you are sensitive to wheat or gluten, you will need to make sure to get gluten-free oats. Buckwheat does not contain wheat or gluten, and barley contains gluten, but not wheat. Healthy beans include any variety you tolerate well.

The key takeaway here is that most people feel healthier when processed grains are removed from their diet. This means cookies, breads, crackers, pastas, etc. Most food that originally started from a grain, and is no longer identifiable as a grain, should be taken out of your diet. Whole grains that are properly soaked and cooked are the healthiest versions to consume.

There are three common themes when it comes to poor grain choices. Of course, the first is choosing processed and refined carbohydrates. Two other troubling trends are:

- The whole-wheat standard American diet is misleading. If you look at the ingredient labels on these products, do you actually see wheat berries (the whole grain) as an ingredient? No, most likely not. You probably see all the wheat parts listed: whole-wheat flour, wheat germ, wheat gluten, and wheat bran. In order for the product to really be whole grain, it needs to say the whole grain in the name. So a whole-wheat product needs to have whole-wheat berries listed as an ingredient. Please do not eat a whole-wheat-based diet of packaged foods; it is not good for your health.

- Gluten-free grains have really made a lot of headway recently. If you are someone who is affected by wheat or gluten, you are probably glad that there are a lot of alternatives lining the shelves these days. Beware, though! Many of these products are just as processed and refined as the refined white (wheat) flour. Sure, it is great to be able to eat a gluten-free pizza sometimes, but remember that to be truly healthy, the grain must be in whole form and properly cooked.

This is why going grain-free can be really healing. However, there is some value to grains and beans, especially as you learn to prepare them appropriately and learn what your body tolerates best. So go ahead and experiment—that is what cooking is all about.

Fats are essential to life. Unfortunately most people are confused about fat. The problem lies in this: fat you eat is not the same thing as adipocytes (body fat). You consume fat and primarily use it as energy; you do not eat fat and automatically store it as fat. When you ingest fat, and it is broken down into fatty acids in the intestine, these fatty acids will be packaged into chylomicrons, which will travel around the body in the blood stream dropping off free fatty acids at tissues to be used for energy. With glucose (sugar), the body will use it for energy as it is in the blood stream, but the moment insulin gets triggered, which is immediately upon consumption of carbohydrates/sugar, the glucose in your blood will immediately begin to be "stored" as insulin is a fat storage hormone.

First the sugar will be stored as glycogen (sugar storage) and then it will be packaged up as triglycerides. This is one main reason why eliminating refined sugar and reducing processed carbohydrates lowers your blood triglyceride lab levels. On the other hand, when you eat fat, you mobilize glucagon, which is the fat breakdown hormone, and this will actually help you "burn energy" and mobilize free fatty acids from the adipocytes to use as fuel. In addition, because fats have more calories per gram than protein or carbohydrates, you feel more full sooner when you eat them. A great tip is to always consume fat with sugar/carbohydrates, as in don't get wrapped up in the no-fat diet, as you will stabilize your blood sugar better if you ingest both fats and carbohydrate sugars together.

Healthy fats include olive oil, coconut oil, butter or ghee (clarified butter), fish oil and cod liver oil, unrefined palm oil, sesame oil, avocado, raw nuts and seeds, and healthy sources of lard. These fats are healthy saturated fats and monounsaturated fats. Unhealthy fats include much of the vegetable oils sold as "healthy" in the conventional healthcare model and nutrition associations. These include canola, corn, soybean, hydrogenated oil, and partially hydrogenated oil. These fats contain more polyunsaturated fatty acid chains, which become rancid more easily and oxidize in your body, causing lipid peroxidation.

QUESTION

Why do I crave salt?
This is common when you have adrenal fatigue, as salt helps to stimulate aldosterone release from the adrenal glands. If you have adrenal fatigue, it is likely that your aldosterone levels are also low. Aldosterone regulates blood pressure and preserves mineral balance in the body. It is released by the same hormone as cortisol, ACTH. As cortisol levels elevate, the brain is signaled to stop releasing ACTH. Eating salt during adrenal fatigue is fine. Your blood pressure most likely needs it. (Salt only negatively impacts about 5 percent of people when it comes to blood pressure.)

The Meal Plan for MSS2–MSS3 versus MSS0–MSS1

When you start to eat healthy meals at the right time of the day, every day, you won't need to think about how many servings of carbohydrates or vegetables you need. You will be eating what you need. Follow the outline for protein, complex carbohydrates, and fats for your level of adrenal fatigue. Use the Meal Plan Checklist in this chapter to make sure you are eating when you should be eating, and use the blood sugar–balancing recipes in this book and refer to other resources to expand your cooking needs. Use snack time to your benefit. Rather than trying to eat some form of sugar or processed carbohydrate, eat protein and vegetables in MSS2–MSS3. In MSS0–MSS1, you probably don't even need snack time. Before you know it, your healthy diet will take on the shape it needs and you will have healed your adrenal fatigue.

The Healthy Meal Plan for MSS0–MSS1

If you are in MSS0–MSS1, or once you heal and transition to this stage of adrenal gland function, you will want to eat more of a ketogenic balanced meal plan that allows you to go into fat-burning mode every day. You will eat less protein, ideally 1gm/kg of protein daily, more quality fats, and complex carbohydrates predominantly in the form of vegetables, with soaked grains and beans as your body can tolerate.

A ketogenic balanced meal plan is a great strategy for long-term health. If you look at your ancestors' lives, you'll see that there were often long times of famine. This meant that the body went into ketosis more regularly, where a majority of the body's energy supply came from ketone bodies due to fat breakdown (lipolysis), as opposed to a state of glycolysis where glucose is the primary energy producer. Most cells in the body can use both glucose and ketone bodies for fuel, and during ketosis, the free fatty acids fuel glucose synthesis (gluconeogenesis in the liver) and this helps meet the remainder of your energy needs. When the body is in ketosis, glucagon (the "fat burning" hormone) circulates more regularly, whereas in glycolysis, insulin (the "fat storage" hormone) circulates predominantly. Thus going into ketosis can be better for more long-term health. Each night when you go to sleep and fast for minimally 8 hours (ideally 12 hours), your body will begin to use fatty acids for fuel. The moment you eat a large carbohydrate meal (bagel, bread, etc.), your body immediately goes back into glycolysis.

Once you move into a stage where your adrenals are mostly healed, you should finish dinner by roughly 3 hours prior to bed. You will go to bed, and your body will burn sugar and then eventually fat for fuel. You have about 6–8 hours of stored sugar as glycogen in the muscle and liver, and your body will use this up first for energy expenditure (yes, even when you sleep you burn energy).

After 8 hours, your body switches to burning fat. So when you wake up, if you can prolong the time you eat breakfast until about 11 A.M., then you have roughly given yourself 8 hours of burning sugar plus another 2–4 hours of fuel burning. If you can do a 25–30 minute cardio workout during this time, then even better. At 10–11 A.M., eat a large meal, ideally the largest of the day.

Then you eat lunch or a snack around 2–3 P.M., and dinner around 6–7 P.M. Please remember, though, that this diet is a ketogenic-balanced routine, and it is *not* ideal for those in MSS2–MSS3,

The Meal Plan Checklist for MSS0–MSS1

❑ If you have relatively healthy adrenals and stress response, then the best dietary guidelines to follow for longevity are for a ketogenic type diet (higher amount of calories from fat). This is not suitable for those in later stages of adrenal fatigue, because blood sugar needs to be more tightly regulated. But for MSS0–MSS1, these individuals can go into fat-burning mode more often and use fat to fuel the body. This means you will not eat breakfast until about 10–11 A.M.

❑ Eat a healthy breakfast around 10–11 A.M. This should be your biggest meal of the day and contain a nice mixture of quality foods coming from vegetables, complex carbs, healthy fats, and protein.

❑ For "lunch" time, you can enjoy a piece of fruit if you still feel hungry (which you shouldn't be if you had a good balance of food for breakfast), or better yet a cup of herbal tea, such as peppermint, holy basil (tulsi), or jasmine green tea—organic, of course.

❑ Eat your second largest meal of the day between 2–3 P.M. This should be a well-balanced meal including veggies, protein, healthy fats, and complex carbs, which can come in the form of vegetable, grain, bean, or nuts and seeds.

❑ Eat a healthy, well-balanced dinner between 5–6:30 P.M. Try to have your dinner be the lightest meal of the day. Homemade soups and bone broths are ideal for this meal and are excellent for your digestive tract.

❑ Generally, if you are in the MSS0–MSS1 stage, you won't need any more food after dinner, though if you have some lingering sleep issues and don't sleep as deeply as you should (and if that is your only health-related complaint), a small piece of protein around 8–8:30 P.M. can help to deepen sleep.

Don't forget to drink your water and healthy beverages between your meals.

The Healthy Meal Plan for MSS2–MSS3

Eating regular meals is important in healing your adrenal glands. Because cortisol regulates blood sugar, when you are in MSS2–MSS3, there are a lot of blood glucose and insulin issues, even if you haven't been officially diagnosed with blood sugar problems. For those in MSS3, your protein needs are most likely the highest because there is so much fatigue. Diets that are heavier in protein during this time are great for healing. You must be careful, though, if you suffer from indigestion, reflux, or low hydrochloric acid, as protein requires adequate acid to be broken down. Some simple ways to improve hydrochloric acid are zinc supplementation, a tablespoon of raw apple cider vinegar in a 12–16-ounce glass of water, or a bitters tincture right before your meal. Eating meals every 2–3 hours is ideal if you are in MSS2–MSS3. Each day you want to eat roughly 1.2gm/kg of protein during this phase. You may even require more protein than this if you are in MSS3, up to 1.3–1.4gm/kg daily.

The Meal Plan Checklist for MSS2–MSS3

❑ Eat breakfast within an hour of getting up, or by no later than 8 A.M., to refresh blood glucose levels that have been depleted overnight. This will also jump-start your metabolism and balance out leptin (the satiety hormone), which will help you have fewer cravings over the day.

One of the big complaints from those who have difficulty losing weight is the pesky adrenal "tire" around the abdomen. If you are someone who has extra weight in your midsection and you are in MSS2–MSS3, then you will want to use breakfast to your advantage in losing weight, by having good-quality protein within 30 minutes of waking. This signals leptin, which is the satiety hormone, and when you eat breakfast while healing adrenal fatigue, you can help keep your leptin level in balance by stimulating the release of it earlier in the day. This actually helps you eat less over the course of the day. Note that you can also burn more fat by eating a ketogenic type diet (higher amount of calories from fat), but most individuals in the more severe forms of adrenal fatigue need more protein and complex carbohydrates to stabilize blood sugar.

- ❑ Eat a healthy snack around 10 A.M., or 2–2½ hours after breakfast. This will keep your blood sugar more stable in the morning time when cortisol levels should be the highest. Snacks should be protein- and vegetable-based.
- ❑ Eat a healthy, balanced lunch around noon to prevent blood sugar from dipping too low, which releases more cortisol.
- ❑ Eat a snack between 2–3 P.M. to offset the natural cortisol dip that occurs around 3–4 P.M. Many people notice this dip every day and reach for extra caffeine or carbohydrate-loaded snacks, which will actually impede hormonal balance.
- ❑ Eat a healthy, well-balanced dinner between 5–6:30 P.M. if you can, and try to have dinner be your lightest meal of the day.
- ❑ Eat a nutritious, light snack an hour before bed to help keep blood sugar levels balanced overnight. Ideally this will be a small piece of protein: 1–2" chunk of cheese, a few tablespoons of yogurt, a teaspoon of almond butter, or a small cup of milk. This protein is not a meal, nor will it be as big as a daytime snack.

Remember to drink your water and healthy beverages between your meals.

Healing the Digestive System

A healthy digestive system is essential to healing the adrenal glands. In fact, a healthy digestive system is a prerequisite for healing any system in the body and maintaining health. Your digestive system is the foundation of your body. It is where you break down and absorb the food that keeps you alive. It is where you absorb the most water, and it is primarily where you excrete waste, toxins, metabolic by-products, etc. A properly functioning digestive system is the base for optimal health.

The Microbiome

Within your digestive system is this amazing balance between letting "good" stuff in and keeping "bad" stuff out. Your stomach has acid in it to kill off pathogens on food so that you don't get sick. Your saliva, pancreas, and gallbladder all work to excrete various substances (enzymes and bile) to improve the breakdown of food, emulsify fats, and set up all nutrients to be properly absorbed.

Your small intestine is the main place where this absorption occurs. Nutrients are brought into the lumen of the small intestine, packaged up, and delivered to the various tissues and organs in the body.

Your large intestine is where you would find the majority of your microbiome (there are also anaerobic bacteria living in the small intestine), which is the amazing plethora of probiotics that help you thrive or, if the wrong kind, can cause serious effects on your health. In fact, there are ten times more microbes in your body than cells.

ESSENTIAL

Probiotics do so much to confer health. Probiotics stimulate the immune system in the gut, turn DNA on and off, help defend the body against invaders, keep your digestive system healthy, turn on and off neurotransmitters, and do so much more.

Your Second Brain

Did you know that your small intestine (aka "your gut") is called the second brain? Do you know why? Your gut has a nervous system of its own, and—even more impressive—over 90 percent of the serotonin made and released in your body comes from your gut, not your brain. However, that serotonin works on your brain, and on all sites that have serotonin receptors. The problem is, what you are eating may not be the right foods to release serotonin when it is needed (for instance tryptophan and vitamin B_6 are needed to make serotonin). In addition, the probiotics living in your digestive system will also influence your serotonin creation and release. Bacteria living in your small intestine actually signal to your intestinal cells to make and release serotonin. So what you eat and how well your digestive system functions (including what lives in your digestive system) will greatly influence your mental and emotional states.

Secretory IgA and Gut Immunity

The third important piece of the digestive system as it relates to adrenal health and whole body health is gut immunity and the secretion of immunoglobulin A (IgA). IgA is secreted in all mucous membranes, including the digestive tract, from mouth to anus. The immunoglobulins are part of the body's "more mature" defense system, and will remember specific pathogens it has been exposed to before. You may be most familiar with IgE, the immunoglobulin responsible for anaphylactic shock. IgA is not necessarily as severe a reaction when stimulated.

Roughly 70 percent of the immune system lives in the digestive tract at a given moment. That is pretty impressive given that the immune system protects the whole body. Again, if you look at the structure and function of the digestive system, it is one of the most likely places a pathogen/invader can interact with the inside of your body. It is imperative that the digestive system be highly supported when it comes to immunity.

In people with adrenal fatigue, lowered immunity is common. This can result in a weaker defense system in the digestive tract, which can manifest locally through digestive symptoms or can translate into more colds, bronchitis, and other respiratory illnesses.

Food Sensitivities, Allergies, and Intolerances

If you feel that food negatively affects you or you experience random symptoms that you have not been able to get answers for, you may suffer from food intolerance or sensitivities. These are different from true allergies, where you eat something and go into anaphylactic shock (IgE). Food sensitivities/intolerances are a delayed type of reaction, known as IgG type reactions. These reactions can take hours to days to show up in the body. People experience varying symptoms from food sensitivities, such as skin conditions, fatigue, brain fog, dark circles under the eyes, allergies, immune challenges, and so on. There are also adverse digestive symptoms that you may experience, such as bloating, constipation, diarrhea, and so forth. You don't have to have digestive symptoms to struggle with food sensitivities—in fact, many people have symptoms in other areas of the body.

If you are curious about food sensitivities, you can get a blood test that will look at IgG levels of common foods. You can also do a simple elimination and challenge diet, where you remove whatever food you suspect is causing you issues for a period of 6 weeks. After 6 weeks, you challenge the food by eating it with each meal for 1–2 days. Now you may feel different right away, and if that is the case, you know this food is bothering you. If you challenge the food and eat it consecutively for 1–2 days and don't feel anything, stop eating it and wait 3–5 days to see if there are any delayed reactions. You can only challenge one food at a time.

CHAPTER 9

Lifestyle Changes

Your lifestyle habits will either make or break your health. You have complete control over what you do in your life, and what habits you create for yourself. Making good lifestyle choices really heals your adrenals and is good for your overall health. Plus, because these lifestyle choices become habits, when you no longer use nutritional therapies your body will have these good practices to fall back on to remain healthy. This is what truly is at the heart of preventative medicine: flipping your disease-promoting habits into health-promoting habits.

Sleep and Your Circadian Rhythm

This is the most fundamental of your healthy lifestyle habits. Why? Your adrenal glands rely on a properly balanced sleep-wake cycle. This means that your overall health relies on a balanced sleep-wake cycle. At the end of the day, if your sleep-wake cycle is disturbed, then your adrenal gland health is disturbed. Your adrenal glands need routine.

So what does a quality sleep-wake cycle look like? Basically, you go to bed, fall asleep in 15–20 minutes, sleep throughout the night, potentially dream, and wake up the next morning after 7½–8½ hours of sleep, ready to start the day. Now, for many people the cycle isn't quite this ironed out. You can begin to improve your sleep-wake cycle by doing the following:

1. Make sure you are getting at least 7–8½ hours of sleep a night depending on your needs: count backwards from the time you have to get up.
2. Make sure your bedroom is pitch-black. Even lights from a TV or alarm clock can disturb the pineal gland in your brain. It doesn't matter whether your eyes are closed or not; if there are lights on in your room, your pineal gland senses it through your skin. Here is a trick: Turn all the lights off in your room and wave your hand in front of your face. If you can see your hand, it is not dark enough.
3. No blue light before bed. What is blue light? Electronics: TV, computer, phones and many hand held electronic devices. Your electronics emit blue light, and this is very stimulating to your body. This light actually suppresses the release of melatonin, and this is why it is so important not to use before bedtime, especially if you have sleep issues. In order to get the best night's sleep you can, you should not watch TV, play on your computer, phone, or gadget, or read an eBook 45–60 minutes before bed. In addition to the blue light, it releases an electromagnetic field, which can also stimulate the body. This is most harmful if you are using a computer, phone, or tablet that sits on your lap or chest because of the close proximity to your body. Instead you can try reading a paper book, meditating, doing a guided visualization, having conversations with loved ones, enjoying some of your own quiet time, journaling, etc.
4. Your room should be cool. Your body will sleep best in a room that is set to 58°F–62°F. If you are having trouble sleeping, try adjusting your room temperature.

5. If you live in a noisy place, you may want to get yourself earplugs. Being woken up, even if you fall back asleep quickly, is still quite disruptive to the natural sleep-wake cycle you are trying to support.

Exercise and Movement

Movement is crucial to your overall health and the health of your adrenal glands. You are meant to move. You are not supposed to sit at a desk all day, nor are you supposed to stand all day. Too much of one activity is not conducive to overall health. Exercise gives you more energy, helps you sleep better, builds bone, keeps your blood sugar and blood pressure in better balance, and much, much more.

Cardiovascular Exercise

When you heal your adrenal glands you also make yourself healthy. Incorporating regular exercise into your health-promoting habits is going to go a long way for your overall health. Cardiovascular exercise does wonders for the health of the sleep-wake cycle and the adrenal glands. High-intensity cardiovascular workouts can be great for health, but you won't want to do more than a 20–25-minute routine if you are attracted to this type of exercise. Those in MSS0–MSS1 will do well with high-intensity exercise. Doing high-intensity cardio more than 20–25 minutes will actually work against you, raising cortisol too much and putting excessive strain on the heart. If you are in MSS2–MSS3, moderate cardiovascular workouts will be good for you, such as biking, brisk walking, hiking, swimming, etc. Moderate exercise can go for longer than 25 minutes, but remember to always listen to your body and only do what it is asking, plus 10 percent, to positively push yourself.

FACT

Exercise is great for both physical and mental health. Here are some of the benefits that exercise has: strengthens your heart, lowers blood pressure, balances blood sugar, builds bone, raises HDL (the "good" cholesterol), improves sleep quality, prevents injuries by increasing muscle strength so that your back and core are strong, improves anxiety, and reduces depression. Those on medications or with health issues are advised to speak with their healthcare provider before starting any new exercise routine.

Weights

It is also beneficial for you to incorporate weights and stretching into your routine. Weights should be used for both upper- and lower-body muscles. You can often use your own weight to create resistance. You can also use resistance bands in your cardio workout, which lets you get your cardio and weight routine in at the same time.

Yoga and Stretching

Lastly, you absolutely need to make stretching or yoga a part of your workout routine. This does not mean taking a 1-hour yoga class once a week. Create a routine. Maybe this means you wake up and stretch and meditate for 20 minutes, or at the end of the day before bed you stretch for 10 minutes. That is much healthier than a 1-hour class four times a month.

Yoga is an ancient Indian tradition of training the physical body to remain fluid and limber, which allows the mind to do the same. There are many different styles of yoga, including hatha, vinyasa, bikram, hot yoga, iyengar, etc. Try taking classes at a local yoga studio and see which style resonates with you. You can also find different yoga styles demonstrated on YouTube, as well as on home DVDs. Stretching and allowing your physical body to remain responsive is really important to your overall physical well-being. The right exercise routine incorporates stretching/yoga as a main component.

Meditation and Mindfulness Practice

Meditation is one of the best fundamental practices you can incorporate into your life, not only to heal your adrenal glands but also to really provide you with a sense of wellness. Meditation is a mindfulness-based practice that allows you to tap into your own mental awareness, struggles, and serenity. You may experience a mind that is full of chatter—most people do. With a regular meditation practice you can quiet your mind, reflect on life, and be able to weather stress. This is not an overnight transformation; it takes consistent work.

All meditation requires is that you be open to spending time in the present moment. These practices are one of the best ways to calm down the mind and spirit, connect with yourself on a deeper level, and connect with your intuition. Next time you eat a meal, try enjoying each bite rather than talking through the entire meal or just shoveling it down. Being mindful of your activities brings a new awareness to what you are doing.

Your mind will most likely be busy every time you try to meditate. The goal is not to sit there with a quiet mind; the goal is to quiet the mind every time a thought appears. The work is done on an ongoing basis. So if you've tried meditating and you've given up because your mind just simply isn't quiet, recognize that the goal is to acknowledge your thoughts and let them go rather than to simply not have them.

Practice is all it takes. Start by sitting for 5 minutes a day and just give yourself the space to let go of thoughts when they arise.

ESSENTIAL

Your daily habits can always be improved upon. Rather than looking at changing your lifestyle to help you heal as "one more thing on your to-do list," you can begin to look at what you are currently doing in your life that may have room for improvement. For instance, if you always have chips or candy for snack time, instead start to bring hummus and cut-up veggie sticks; if you skip exercise for TV, try getting yourself a workout DVD for home and committing to 2 days a week. Once you have some good habits established, you will naturally be inclined to add more of them as you see the benefits.

Sense of Purpose

Being connected to something bigger than yourself will allow you to find hope when you feel like there is none. Knowing that you are not alone can help you fulfill a deeper need within your soul. You are here for a reason, whatever it may be; only you and your higher self know. Having a sense of purpose allows you to do all those things such as find hope, power through, or continue on, even during those times when you feel that you could just give up.

You should always strive to understand what that is. In order for you to continually evolve as an individual, you have a physical, mental, and spiritual side of yourself that will always want to live, learn, and grow. Helping your adrenal glands stay healthy will require that you be connected to your purpose. Connecting to your purpose will allow those stressful moments to roll right off of you.

Let Go, You're Not in Control

Whether you realize it or not, you are not in control. You can experience moments of having control, such as paying your bills on time, ordering what you would like at a restaurant, choosing the man of your dreams, or strategically planning out when you will have a child. But think back over your life, and remember those times when the people you love did what they wanted rather than what you wanted them to do.

When you want to have control over every aspect of your life, and you don't, this often brings up feelings of anxiety. You may feel anxiety differently than someone else. For instance, you may feel tightness in your chest, or have difficulty breathing including shallow breathing or hyperventilating; you may feel jumpy, experience a scattered mind, have to pace, or feel irritable. Any of these feelings may arise because you are "not in control."

If reading this creates strong reaction (positive or negative), then this is something you will want to address. Committing to some of the practices within this book will definitely provide you with some relief. However, what you really will need to do is accept that you do *not* have control over every situation.

Connect with Nature

Getting outside can be one of the best ways to heal your adrenal glands. Connecting with Mother Nature is extremely healing to the body, mind, and spirit. Your adrenals are part of the circadian rhythm that nature produces. Think about it: When the sun comes up, you wake up with the sun and your cortisol levels should be the highest. As the sun goes down over the course of the day, so do your cortisol levels. And as the moon rises, it is time for you to retire for bed and get a good night's sleep.

When you get outside, you experience fresh air on your skin and air in your lungs. This is one of the best ways to ground your emotions. Do some deep breathing outdoors when you feel anxious, irritable, or overwhelmed. Having the sun hit your skin (when it is sunny out) provides you with vitamin

D. Having your feet planted on the bare earth, whether in shoes or not, allows you to stabilize your emotional and mental energy.

One of the best ways to reconnect with yourself, your "why" and purpose, is to get out in nature, clear your head, let go of your to-do list, do some deep breathing, and just take in the world around you. You are sure to feel inspired and creative after doing this.

If you experience stage 2 or 3 adrenal fatigue, one of the best activities you can do to re-regulate your HPA axis is to go outside for 30 minutes right after you wake up. This may require some bundling up depending on the time of year, but even in the winter, this therapy does a lot for normalizing the sleep-wake cycle. Getting natural light onto your body and fresh air into your lungs will help your adrenal glands understand that it is morning time, and that cortisol levels should be at their highest. This is best done daily. If you experience stage 0 or stage 1 adrenal fatigue, this practice is most definitely beneficial for all.

Earthing and Grounding

Earthing is a grounding practice that involves you walking on the earth barefoot. Through this practice there is great potential for you to connect to your body, mind, and spirit and to the earth, which many people believe helps to ground them and provide them with a sense of serenity. Obviously this may not always be possible depending on where you live and what time of year it is. So, you also can perform earthing by buying a special pad designed to simulate the earth's electromagnetics.

QUESTION

Are you affected by anxiety?
Anxiety disorders are the most common mental illness in the United States, affecting 20 percent of adults, with another 20 percent of adults being affected by anxiety at some point in their life. If you are trying to get control of your anxiety, here are some things for you to try: deep breathing, question your thoughts, accept that you feel anxious, use positive self-talk, focus on the moment as well as meaningful activities, and observe your thoughts and feelings rather than judging them.

Most of the research on earthing is preliminary, but shows promise in the following effects on the body and mind: reducing cortisol and self-perceived stress, improving sleep, reducing electromagnetic frequency stimulation, and helping to shift the autonomic nervous system from sympathetic dominance to parasympathetic. The sympathetic nervous system is the one activated in the fight-or-flight reaction.

Deep Breathing

Breathing is vital to life, so vital that you don't even have to consciously think about doing it. Slow and deep breathing reduces dead space between the inspiration and expiration cycle of the lungs, and allows for better transfer of oxygen with carbon dioxide. Pranayama, a practice of deep breathing originating from India as part of the yogic tradition, has long demonstrated beneficial effects. In a 2011 study in the *Indian Journal of Physiology and Pharmacology* (*IJPP*), researchers looked at pulmonary function tests after deep breathing in healthy volunteers. Researchers found that even short-duration deep breathing, as little as 2–5 minutes, significantly improves one's ability to get carbon dioxide out of the lungs, and allowed for better oxygen intake upon the next inspiration.

In a 2012 study, also in the *IJPP*, researchers looked at the effect of deep breathing on heart rate variability in healthy volunteers. This time, volunteers were randomized for daily deep-breathing exercises for one month. Researchers found that simple deep breathing had a positive effect on cardiac autonomic modulation, meaning that deep-breathing exercises improved heart rate variability without stimulating an imbalance in the sympathetic-parasympathetic balance of the heart. Heart rate variability is important for long-term heart health. You want your heart rate to vary the amount of beats it has per minute rather than consistently beat at the same moment every single moment of your life. Improved heart rate variability means that your heart is better able to adapt to stressors.

Get Started Today

Deep-breathing exercises often amount to 5–6 deep breaths per minute. Sit down with a stopwatch and do 5 minutes of deep breathing, with 6 breaths per minute. As you practice, you won't need to watch each minute, as you will become familiar with your rate of breathing. As you go, set yourself a 10–15-minute alarm and sit down to do some deep breathing. This is the perfect activity to bring into other parts of your life: at a meeting, sitting in traffic, during a heated discussion.

Reiki

Reiki is a Japanese technique for stress reduction and relaxation that promotes healing. The therapist channels energy into the patient by means of touch, activating the natural healing processes of the patient's body and allowing for restoration of physical and emotional well-being. Reiki is taught by Reiki masters who tap into "life force energy" to be able to transfer it to the client.

In the journal *Biological Research for Nursing*, a 2011 study looked at the effects of Reiki on twenty-one healthcare professionals who experienced burnout relating to their work. Participants underwent two Reiki sessions 1 week apart. The active group was given Reiki by an experienced individual and the other received "placebo" sessions from someone who never trained in Reiki but followed the same flow as the experienced Reiki practitioner. The results were significant and demonstrated that Reiki had a calming effect on the parasympathetic nervous system, by improving ECG readings, as well as increasing body temperature.

Healing touch with guided imagery (HT+GI) has also been studied in post-traumatic stress disorder (PTSD), which is a condition with many similar findings as adrenal fatigue when it comes to cortisol's effects on the brain. Active duty military were selected to receive 6 weeks of sessions, and a statistically and clinically significant difference was noted in PTSD symptoms as well as depression in those who underwent HT+GI therapy. There was also a trend toward improvement in mental clarity and a reduction in cynicism.

Tai Chi

Tai chi is an ancient Chinese form of self-defense. Today, it is practiced as a graceful form of exercise, providing a moderate level of aerobic exercise while inducing a meditative state. It is often referred to as "meditation in motion," as it promotes a sense of calmness through a series of flowing movements accompanied by deep breathing.

In experimental studies, tai chi practice is associated with an elevation in heart rate and an increased excretion of urinary norepinephrine, decreased salivary cortisol, less mood disturbance, a reduced state of anxiety, and increased feelings of vigor. A 1992 study found that tai chi, brisk walking, and meditation resulted in a statistically significant decrease in salivary cortisol and an overall improvement in mood states across each treatment group. The tai chi group also had an elevation in heart rate comparable to the brisk-walking group, suggesting that tai chi's stress-reducing ability was due to similar effects as moderate exercise.

Additional Ways to Support Adrenal Gland Healing

You have learned a number of lifestyle habits that you can begin today to start healing your adrenal glands. Don't try to do everything at once; this often leads to failure. Instead pick 1–2 new lifestyle habits you want to incorporate into your life. Start with just a 5–10-minute practice for each, and once they become habits, move on to the next thing. Before you know it, you will have flipped your disease-promoting habits into health-promoting habits. Here are some additional lifestyle habits that will help balance your adrenal glands and HPA axis for long-term health:

- Laughter on a daily basis
- Alone time—just as important as connecting with loved ones and friends
- Journaling, writing, or being creative, including art
- Friends, making time for the people who are special in your life
- Play-time, not just for kids—everyone needs some time to just let go

- Sunshine in the morning: if you are in MSS2–MSS3, one of the best things to do is to get outside as soon as you wake up to re-regulate your sleep-wake cycle, even on cold days

The Importance of Detoxification (Supporting Elimination)

Supporting the natural detoxification channels in your body is one of the best ways to promote optimal health. Your body is detoxifying as you read these pages, so going on a detox one or two times a year is really not the best strategy for long-term health. Yes, you can get some short-term benefits from doing this, but if you're not using your diet and lifestyle as well as natural therapies to support detoxification year-round, then you are not fully supporting a healthy body.

When you think of detox, you may think of bowel elimination or having your skin break out. Many detox routines and regimens push detox pathways hard, making the body's natural detox pathways overwhelmed and bogged down. Why not take the approach of gently supporting these pathways all the time so that you are getting rid of waste and toxins every day and not overburdening or overwhelming your system? The last thing you want is to cause secondary symptoms because you pushed detoxification pathways when your five primary pathways of detox were not optimally set up to clear the waste out.

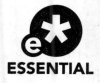

ESSENTIAL

Detoxification is an essential part of being alive. Your body is detoxifying every moment of every day. Here are a list of symptoms that you may experience if your detoxification processes are overburdened: fatigue, sluggish bowel habits, irritated skin or regular skin blemishes, allergies, mental fog or lack of focus, puffy eyes, circles or bags under the eyes, bloating, PMS or menstrual complaints, joint aches not due to a specific condition, or headaches.

Five Pathways

The five pathways are the digestive tract and liver, kidneys, lungs, skin, and emotions. Your body already has these natural pathways of elimination to get rid of waste and toxins from both internal metabolic pathways and externally from chemicals you are exposed to on a daily basis. The goal is to support these pathways every single day, and you will do that by flipping your disease-promoting habits into health-promoting habits.

Why is this important for adrenal health? When your body is overwhelmed with metabolic and chemical waste, this is a major stressor on your system. Reducing the burden of chemicals will allow the body to be more efficient at staying healthy and will give your adrenal glands a rest from worrying about what metabolic pathways are not functioning optimally. Start by adding some of the following habits into your daily life, all of which support various pathways of elimination in your body:

- Drinking lemon water in the morning will help wake up your digestive system and the liver. It is a very gentle detoxifier of the liver and adds a good dose of bioflavonoids to the diet. Use 8–10 ounces of water and the juice of ¼–½ lemon depending on taste preference.
- Dry skin brushing is a wonderful way to stimulate the superficial lymphatics. This therapy helps promote movement of the lymph, which is responsible for moving waste to appropriate areas for removal from the body, as well as carrying parts of your immune system around, such as macrophages and neutrophils, so that should a pathogen get inside the body, the lymphatic system has immune cells ready to launch a defense. Should backup be needed, those cells will send signals to the rest of the immune system.
- Castor oil packs are commonly done over the abdomen and are a deeper lymphatic therapy, excellent for healing the digestive system. Use at least 4 days a week to get the best benefits of moving waste to the liver and digestive system to be excreted.
- Sweating regularly, at least 3 days a week but ideally every day, can be done through many avenues, including exercise, sauna, steam, or a hot bath/shower. Promoting detoxification through the skin via sweating and opening the pores is one of the best and safest ways to detox.
- Getting fresh oxygen daily allows the body to meet its needs for this vital molecule and helps you use your lungs to get rid of waste in the form of

carbon dioxide, keeping the body in a good acid-alkaline balance. Getting out of indoor environments regularly is ideal, as these manmade areas are often full of chemicals.

- Getting outdoors daily and getting sunlight is a twofold strategy. In addition to getting you fresh oxygen, going outdoors also gives you sun on your skin, which is an amazing medicine for your body and mind.

- Having a way to let go of emotions is crucial to healing and supporting the adrenal glands. One of the most common reasons for adrenal fatigue/hypoadrenia is a major grief. This will also affect the lungs, as, according to Chinese medicine, the lungs are the organ related to grief and sadness. You can process and let go of emotions through various means, including getting outside and connecting with nature, journaling, deep breathing, talking with someone, or crying. All of these will help—and you may even have your own way that you already process your emotions, so use that too!

- Connecting with yourself daily is key to transforming your health. You are a spiritual being who is being challenged every day to grow physically, mentally, emotionally, and spiritually. This is not religion. This is being alive. However, what you use may be different from what someone else uses to connect daily. For you it may be religious, surrounding yourself with nature, going for a hike, or doing mindfulness mediation.

- Mindfulness practices are essential to helping you break through the inherent challenges you will face on a daily basis as a human being. This will help keep the emotions and the mind able to detox regularly by allowing you to feel more centered and able to check in with your emotions; letting go of them with the aid of a journal may help. Becoming more mindful allows you to assess what you are holding onto that may be ready for letting go.

- Drinking adequate clean water is essential to life. At this point, unless you live in a place where you can find clean water, you will probably want to filter yours. You want to remove chlorine, fluoride, and the myriad of pharmaceuticals that show up in water in most communities. Water keeps the kidneys and skin able to get rid of waste and helps hydrate the body to function optimally, leaving you with clear skin, strong hair, balanced blood pressure and blood volume, and much more.

- Eating lots of fresh vegetables is a great way to make sure you get plenty of nutrients, especially vitamins and minerals, as well as water on a daily basis.

- Eating good-quality fats is necessary to help your body burn fat. Your fat stores are burned when you eat fat and the new fat you eat replaces older fat regularly. This includes cell membrane fats. You also store most toxins in your fat. After all, your body is smart. If it can't get rid of toxins and waste, it needs to put it somewhere, so into your fat (and bones) it goes. However, this isn't really a great long-term strategy.
- Infrared sauna improves sweating and allows the body to detox through the skin. You can check out the resources for ways to incorporate this into your home life if you can't find a facility near you that offers it.

ALERT

While the lymphatic system often takes a backseat to other "more important" systems such as the cardiovascular system, many countries worldwide recognize the importance of this system to the health of so many other systems in the body including the immune, digestive, nervous, circulatory ,and detoxification systems, and recommend therapies to support it. Your lymphatic system is made up of lymph nodes, lymph vessels, your spleen and thymus, GALT and BALT (gut-associated lymphoid tissue and bronchus-associated lymphoid tissue), and your tonsils.

Putting It All Together

A healthy lifestyle is the best way you can accelerate healing on a daily basis—not only of your adrenal glands, but of your whole body. Start with one new practice a month. The goal is to make it stick as part of your routine. If you have never tried some of the recommendations here, go search them out in your community or through the resources section. Be flexible in your mind and allow yourself the opportunity to try new things. If you fail, get up and try again. The goal with your lifestyle changes is to make regular deposits to the adrenal bank account, so that when you do undergo stressors or a major stressful event, you have these lifestyle habits to fall back on to provide a resiliency, recovery, and plenty of deposits in the account. You deserve the healthiest life you can have, so go out and get it.

CHAPTER 10

The Many Faces of Healing Adrenal Fatigue

The primary focus of this book is healing the HPA axis through the right diet, lifestyle factors, and natural therapies. Of course, you may see that there are additional areas in your body that need to be treated alongside the adrenals. Your adrenals affect nearly all other systems in your body. While you are healing your adrenals, other systems that are showing symptoms will need to be healed as well in order for your adrenals to fully heal. Some of these symptoms will get better as a result of your improved adrenal health, and others will require distinctive support.

Healing Adrenal Fatigue with Quality Natural Therapies

The nutritional supplements you use to heal your adrenal glands are completely dependent on what your adrenal hormones are telling you through lab work and what symptoms you currently have or have recently experienced. Your past medical history, family medical history, as well as your quality of life (diet, lifestyle, work, social, environmental history) and your standard bloodwork are also all great tools to use to find out what triggered the adrenal fatigue. A good health history will give you a lot of information on what additional systems need healing, and this will be important when addressing your adrenal fatigue.

Start with assessing your adrenal health before you go and try to buy the best supplements to support your adrenals. Try not to just buy the newest fad when it comes to supplements, and make sure you understand what the product will do for your adrenals, hormones, and nervous system. The best thing you can do is start by getting your adrenal hormones tested using a variable salivary test, so that you don't inadvertently go buy something intended for overactive adrenal gland function when in fact you have under-functioning adrenal glands!

Support for a Mostly Healthy Adrenal System (MSS0)

Your adrenal gland system is designed to respond to stress, and then help you return to a balanced state. This is healthy and normal. In order to keep yourself balanced in the stressful world you live in, there are specific therapies you can use as needed.

Generally, it is good to have these therapies on hand, depending on your personal constitution, the season of the year, and the activities you have going on. This is what is called preventative medicine. When you are relatively healthy, you don't want to assume you will stay healthy as you age; you want to be proactive about keeping yourself healthy. If you have few to no symptoms and you want to prevent the heart disease your dad's family has or the diabetes rampant in your mother's family, then preventative medicine, which includes keeping your stress response and adrenal glands healthy, is the way to go.

Nutrients such as the antioxidants vitamin A, vitamin C, vitamin E, and zinc are all useful therapies when your body is under increased stress. Say you have a lot of kids' activities going on, have a few big projects at work due, or are trying to stay healthy while those around you have symptoms of the cold. Vitamin C is great for cold and flu season, as your adrenals concentrate vitamin C and your HPA axis will need to respond when others around you are sick (being exposed to illness is a stressor).

Herbal remedies are a great therapy to have on hand to use preventatively or as needed. For instance, if you tend to sleep lightly, ashwagandha is a great herbal adaptogen to add to your bedtime routine. This herb will help you sleep better, which is perfect for the adrenal system, and will give you optimal energy during the day.

QUESTION

Why is it so important to get a good night's sleep in healing adrenal gland function?
Remember that your daytime energy levels depend on your depth and quality of sleep. The better you sleep, and the more restorative your sleep is, the better your body will heal and repair overnight. The adrenal glands, as well as the entire endocrine system, are busy at night repairing the body and getting it ready for the coming day. The deeper the sleep, the better the repair process, and the better your energy levels the following day.

Another great herbal adaptogen to use preventatively is holy basil (tulsi). This is great to use as a morning or mid-afternoon tea on a daily basis. It will give you energy, but not stimulate you; it will help you feel more whole-body nourished, grounded, and calm, which is a combination unique to this herb and different from the effects of other herbs that support the adrenal gland system.

If you tend to get a bad cold each year, or just have lower energy from raising a family or being busier than you would like, the ginsengs are great herbs to support you. There is American ginseng and Asian ginseng. They are both stimulating and energizing to the body; however, Asian ginseng is much more stimulating than American.

As you read through the therapies to heal the stages of adrenal fatigue, you may also find that some of them speak to how you feel some days or could possibly help treat symptoms you occasionally experience. These therapies can often be used as needed or in a preventative health routine, such as a B-complex vitamin for times when you are under greater stress. You are unique; find what works best for you.

Healing MSS1

The defining factor in MSS1 is that there has not been an appropriate recovery period from acute stressors. The adrenal gland system is still responding in the normal fashion of increasing output when you experience stress, but you are not returning to a state of homeostasis after the stress is no longer there. Your brain still believes the stress is there, and you don't have enough reserves in your adrenal bank account or you incur too many stressors too close together. Thus the body doesn't completely recover.

Healing MSS2

Hyperadrenia is the main cause of symptoms in this stage. The adrenal glands have been asked to respond to stressors over and over again, and are now in an elevated state of output of adrenal hormones. There are two different ways you may respond: you may be the stressed and wired type (inability to calm down) or the stressed and worried type (inability to focus). You may experience some of both.

The therapies used in handling this stage of adrenal fatigue generally help calm down the adrenal glands, help the brain and nervous system be able to better focus, and support the HPA axis. This is why it is vitally important for you to know what your adrenal gland hormone output looks like on labs before you start treating yourself for adrenal fatigue.

If you were to use one of the ginsengs as an adaptogen in this phase, you would overstimulate an already stimulated system. Please, do not just go out and buy the hottest new trend to heal your adrenal glands (or anything). Try to switch your mind from "I'm going to get a pill in a bottle and that will cure me" to "I'm going to do the work of flipping my disease-promoting habits into health-promoting habits using my diet and lifestyle and natural therapies to heal my adrenals sustainably." You will have much better long-term results with the latter. This stage requires longer-term treatment and various therapies to heal symptoms in other areas of the body.

Healing MSS3

The final stage of adrenal fatigue is the one commonly referred to as hypoadrenia or adrenal burnout. This stage can be a culmination of constant stresses on the body with little to no recovery between stressors, the result of an inadequate adrenal bank account to support the adrenals in doing their job, or the aftermath of one major life event.

This stage will take more time to heal, and may often require more therapies starting out. Like stage 2, this stage often has symptoms in various systems, and will therefore require a long-term strategy for treatment. You may experience stress with mental fatigue, stress with physical fatigue, or most likely some combination of both.

Nutritional Supplements to Heal Adrenal Fatigue

The primary goal is to heal the adrenal glands using diet and lifestyle, stress management techniques, and a healthy routine as the foundation of treatment, using appropriate natural therapies to support and accelerate the healing process. Once the adrenal glands and the HPA axis have healed, using only the supplements that are needed for preventative medicine and foundational support should keep the system in balance. Of course, you always have these therapies to turn to should a major stressor disrupt your progress.

The most important piece of information you need to know about buying supplements is the following: you must read ingredients of all supplements you purchase. Do not expect that because the front says "highly absorbable," "natural," or "organic" that the bottle really lives up to that truth. You must know what you are taking. Read all ingredients, which means turn the bottle around and read the nutrition label. What ingredients are you putting into your body? Be trusting, but also retain some healthy skepticism.

The second most valuable piece of information you need to know is that you get what you pay for. If you shop based only on price, expect to get low quality.

ESSENTIAL

If you want to take the best care of your health, you need to understand what you are putting into your body. Most importantly, if you are going to treat yourself, you need to know if any supplements interact poorly with anything else. This is imperative when mixing pharmaceuticals with natural therapies. Natural is generally safer, but understanding the dose, quality, and interactions are all vital.

Many people want to try to heal themselves. It is a lot of trial and error. This is why an individualized treatment from a knowledgeable healthcare professional can go a long way. You are more than welcome to educate yourself on what the best therapy is for you, but remember that you need to do your homework. Reading one blog, or one book, or watching a TV show on natural medicine is not going to be enough for you to heal your adrenal glands if you suffer from MSS2 or MSS3 adrenal fatigue. In these stages, there are multiple interactions of symptoms in various systems, which require insight, forethought, and due diligence to understand how to heal the system and the whole body. If you are in stage 0 or stage 1 and just trying to support your adrenal gland system with some specific natural therapies, then you may be able to get away with doing less homework.

The therapies that follow are the most common therapies used in the restoration of adrenal gland health and the HPA axis. There are many other therapies that you may need, depending on your unique physiology, medical history, genetics, and more. This information is a good place to start when healing your adrenal glands. A comprehensive approach to treatment often involves the use of nutritional therapies as needed, and then removing the therapeutic supplements as the adrenal glands and stress response heal. The basics of diet and lifestyle will keep the adrenal gland system healed once the therapeutics have been removed.

Evaluating Your Nutritional Supplements

The supplement industry is not well regulated and there are many products out there (a large majority) whose quality is quite low. If you have no response to treatment, it may also mean that you have not picked out an effective supplement brand. Make sure you buy products that were developed by companies that have qualified healthcare professionals in the Science and Innovation/R&D departments.

Supplements that just lead to energy surges may actually be quite dangerous to an individual suffering from MSS3 adrenal fatigue. You want to make sure that your response to treatment is safe and effective for restoring health, not just alleviating symptoms. Of course, you want to relieve symptoms as well, but the real goal is to nourish and heal the adrenal glands with natural therapies. Once recovered, you can continue to use the transformed diet and lifestyle, along with a few choice natural therapies, to maintain adrenal gland health. You deserve the best in your recovery, so make sure you get it.

Nutritional Therapies and Your Response

Remember that your optimum therapeutic dose may be quite different from someone else's, even someone at the same level of adrenal fatigue. Dosages given here are guidelines. The only way to know what levels will work best for you is to do research. Your response to treatment will also give you information. If you respond negatively to something, it may mean that other biochemical pathways have not been well supported, or that your dose is too high, or that you simply don't need that nutrient at this time.

You can also expect differences in how nutrients affect you at varying levels. For instance, vitamin C at a high dose, as well as magnesium, may cause loosening of stools. While this may be advantageous for someone who also experiences constipation, the dose is too much for individuals who don't need that type of support. Vitamin C is also a main antioxidant in the body, and those who have more chemical storage may experience a surge of "toxicity" type symptoms (headaches, loose stools, skin rashes) if too much is added or additional supportive therapies are not concomitantly used.

Vitamins for Adrenal Gland Health

The following is a list of vitamins that help heal your adrenals. Each has its own special purpose, and will deliver specific results.

Vitamin B$_5$ (Pantothenic Acid)

Vitamin B$_5$ helps to convert food into fuel (glucose) for energy; it is crucial for the production of red blood cells and it supports the creation of sex and steroid hormones. Vitamin B$_5$ also supports digestive function and wound healing, and aids the body in using other B vitamins, specifically B$_2$, riboflavin. B$_5$ can be found in a wide variety of foods, but is often lost with processing. With pantothenic acid (look for that on labels), 40–250mg two times a day may be used. The dose depends on severity of symptoms and what other conditions you have; higher doses (in grams) are often used with more severe adrenal fatigue.

Vitamin B$_3$ and Vitamin B$_6$

These vitamins are crucial for supporting healthy hormone production, including cortisol, as well as supporting metabolic (energy production from food) and detoxification pathways in the body. These vitamins work as enzymes keeping the cholesterol moving forward to generate all the adrenal and sex hormones. The dosage for vitamin B$_3$ (niacin) is 75–150mg daily. You may need less or more, depending on your other complaints with your adrenal fatigue symptoms (niacin and inositol hexanicotinate are more implicated in blood cholesterol balancing, whereas niacinamide is more implicated in blood sugar regulation). Niacin can cause flushing, so niacinamide and inositol hexanicotinate are better utilized for many in the treatment of adrenal fatigue.

The dosage for vitamin B$_6$ (pyridoxine) is 50–300mg daily, depending on severity and personal need. This vitamin supports the creation of cortisol and allows for cortisol to act as a glucocorticoid (blood sugar regulator). Often a B-complex, which provides all the B vitamins in one product, can be good for those with MSS0–MSS1 who experience stress, whereas those in MSS2–MSS3 may need higher dosages of particular B vitamins.

Vitamin B$_{12}$

Vitamin B$_{12}$ (methylcobalamin, adenosylcobalamin, hydroxocobalamin) is often used for adrenal fatigue because of its role in nervous system support. B$_{12}$ assists in mitochondrial function and energy production of the cell. Methylcobalamin is a methyl donor, and supports a healthy methylation cycle. Those with a genetic defect in the MTHFR gene may find that more methylcobalamin is needed to help support the body. Vitamin B_{12} can be taken orally, sublingually (under the tongue), and through an injection. Using the oral method is the most difficult in terms of absorption, because vitamin B_{12} requires healthy quantities of hydrochloric acid and intrinsic factor from the stomach. As a note, please stay away from cyanocobalamin. This is a cheap form of cobalamin (vitamin B_{12}) and your body must get rid of the cyanide molecule.

Vitamin C and Vitamin E

Vitamin C and accompanying bioflavonoids are crucial in adrenal cascade/hormone production. Adrenocorticotropic hormone (ACTH) causes the adrenals to release stored vitamin C to produce cortisol. During times of adrenal fatigue, the adrenals may be so weak that the release of vitamin C is insufficient or overly exaggerated, in an attempt to make more cortisol and adrenal hormones. Vitamin C is water-soluble, so it must be ingested regularly through the diet and supplements. Vitamin C from supplements is almost always derived from corn, which can be difficult if you have an allergy. Vitamin C also supports the immune system, including antimicrobial and natural killer cell activities (protect against cancerous cells), lymphocyte production, migration of cells across tissues, and delayed-type hypersensitivity (IgG—immunoglobulin G).

The more severe the adrenal fatigue, the higher the dose of vitamin C that is often needed. Signs of vitamin C deficiency are: swollen or sore gums, bleeding during tooth brushing, and easy bruising. Vitamin C, alongside antioxidants such as vitamin E, will help to reduce oxidative stress formed naturally in the body when cells are busy working. For the adrenal glands, reactive oxygen species are generated when lots of cortisol is continually being produced. Many people with adrenal fatigue and symptoms of exhaustion benefit from starting a 500–1000mg regimen of vitamin C daily. Vitamin C, like magnesium, has a laxative effect, so you may want to dose yourself up by 500mg each day until you reach bowel tolerance (develop loose stools) and back down by 500mg. For those with severe adrenal fatigue, sometimes 3–5 grams (3000–5000mg) of vitamin C is needed in the recovery phase. Vitamin C is not indicated for those with hyperadrenia. This stage of adrenal fatigue often has elevated cortisol levels, and vitamin C promotes cortisol production and increases the half-life of cortisol, which slows its breakdown allowing for more cortisol to circulate in the body. While you do not have to limit vitamin C in your diet (you still need vitamin C for health), often a vitamin C supplement for stage 2 is not necessary. As you heal, this may change.

Vitamin E is essential to adrenal health, as it acts as an antioxidant. Vitamin E enhances vitamin C's ability to act as a free radical–scavenging agent, so it acts as an antioxidant and helps recycle vitamin C for more antioxidant activity. When looking to purchase vitamin E in a supplement, you definitely want to make sure you are getting a mixed tocopherol product. Originally alpha-tocopherol was the only one isolated, and it is actually problematic to take alpha without the other tocopherols, negatively influencing cardiovascular health. 400IU daily of a mixed tocopherol is a great addition, especially if you suffer from much oxidative stress and/or cardiovascular issues.

Minerals for Adrenal Gland Health

The following is a list of minerals you can take to support and heal your adrenal glands. Minerals are necessary for many biochemical reactions in the body and support nearly all systems. This is not an exhaustive list of minerals, but these are the more common ones used when healing the adrenal glands and supporting the body during times of stress.

Magnesium

Magnesium is generally found in the soil and is delivered on our food and in our food. However, the use of depleted soils and the washing of produce has created a situation where little magnesium is left on the vegetables. While you can still get magnesium from the vegetable itself, you get less total overall magnesium from the diet today than your ancestors got. This is why magnesium is a good mineral to get in a supplement. Three out of four people don't even get the RDA (Recommended Daily Allowance) of magnesium, and the RDA may not even be enough for you if you are not healthy.

Magnesium comes in many different forms, and most of them have laxative effects, though this varies depending on the type. Magnesium citrate is highly absorbable, and often has the strongest laxative effect and muscle-relaxing effect. Magnesium taurate and glycinate are often used in treatment where cardiovascular support is needed. Magnesium malate supports ATP generation and can be really helpful along with citrate for adrenal fatigue. Magnesium chloride can best support detoxification pathways.

FACT

Magnesium is responsible for hundreds of biochemical reactions in the body. Magnesium supports digestion, reproduction, the musculoskeletal system, the brain and nervous system, energy levels, the health of the adrenals, and the detoxification of heavy metals. You are unlikely to get enough magnesium from your diet, so a supplement is often a good idea.

There are various forms of delivery of magnesium as well. Most of the previously mentioned forms of magnesium supplements are taken orally, but there are other therapies including Epsom salts baths (sulfate) and topical magnesium sprays (often chloride).

A good dose of magnesium is between 200–500mg daily. This is a ballpark range and will suffice for many. Depending on the type of magnesium you buy, you may need less (if too much laxative effect) or more, often up to 700–800mg (total from diet and supplement) if you have stage 3 adrenal fatigue, where you are in burnout. Again, you are an individual, so make sure to play with dosages and read all the ingredients on the brand you buy so you know you are getting the right type for what your body needs.

Calcium

Calcium supports adrenal gland health by acting as a stress absorber for the body when a stressor hits. It initiates adrenal hormone secretion, helping relay messages through the nervous and endocrine systems and acts to help muscles appropriately contract and relax. A dose of 500–1000mg daily of a citrate-malate is desirable if your symptoms point to calcium support. Calcium should never be used on its own, because it requires other co-factors to help get it to where it needs to be in the body (in the muscles and bones). It is always good to make sure your calcium supplement has magnesium, vitamin D, vitamin K_1 and K_2, and minerals such as boron and strontium.

Trace Minerals

Zinc, iron, selenium, copper, molybdenum, manganese, iodine, chromium, boron, lithium, and vanadium are all trace minerals that your body needs. You may need more of one than another. The type of trace minerals you may need depends on your symptoms. The best forms to get these trace minerals in are glycinate chelate or picolinate form. Good sources of iodine can often be found as iodide or kelp.

If you have immune and/or digestive issues, then zinc may be helpful. If you have thyroid issues, both selenium and iodine may be needed. Your body may need more of one trace mineral than another, depending on your phase of life as well. Women who are pregnant may need adequate levels of iodine to help a developing fetus's brain health, as well as her own thyroid health.

Manganese, zinc, and potassium are all crucial to steroid hormone and adrenal gland function. They are the main minerals responsible for these enzymatic reactions in this area of the body. Remember that biochemical reactions (which make up your body) are all facilitated and supported by enzymes and substrates. Substrates are the raw materials such as cholesterol, whereas enzymes are often the nutrients, vitamins, and minerals in your food. In order for a reaction to occur (for example, the creation of cortisol), both substrate and enzymes are needed to successfully complete the process. For the adrenals, manganese, potassium, and zinc are all vital.

In addition, being deficient in any of these minerals will cause a physiologic stress on the body that will in turn require more adrenal gland output. Minerals can be found in either liquid or capsule form; they can also be applied to the skin, used in baths, or taken orally. Generally minerals from the sea or salt pools are the best, as these are naturally occurring and the sea's mineral content mirrors what our blood's plasma mineral ratio looks like.

CHAPTER 11

Healing Adrenal Fatigue and MSS1–MSS3 Treatment Protocols

Healing the adrenal glands requires a clear and very well thought out treatment protocol. What works for some stages will not work for others. Your dose and response to treatment will be uniquely your own. You will at times feel overwhelmed by information, but remember to start slowly and add in one new thing at a time. The diet and lifestyle pieces are the most crucial, and the nutritional therapies will be much more effective in your treatment with a strong foundation of dietary and lifestyle practices, as well as health-promoting habits.

Herbal Medicine for Adrenal Gland Health

Herbs are one of the very best therapies to use for both the maintenance and restoration of health. Herbs are wonderful, because the medicine can be extracted by making a strong infusion or decoction or by using a medium such as alcohol, honey, or apple cider vinegar to extract the medicine.

Herbs, like humans, can constitutionally run hot, warm, or cold. If you are someone who is always cold, a warming herb is going to serve you best. You will notice that some herbs are drying, which often coincides with warming, while others are moistening, which often goes with cooling tendencies. If you are someone who experiences hot flashes or irritability, you may do better with cooler herbs.

Adaptogens

These herbs are wonderful at helping you cope, calming you down if necessary, energizing you if necessary, and promoting resistance and resilience, as well as supporting your immune system, which is your primary defense. Each adaptogen may do something different, depending on what your body needs.

You will find that some adaptogens give you stimulating energy. If you are in MSS2, the last thing you need is more stimulation; you actually need to calm your adrenals and HPA axis. If you are in MSS0–MSS1 or MSS3, specific adaptogens can provide you with some sustainable energy that keeps you from burning out your adrenals. Most adaptogens energize you in a very restorative, nonstimulating way. The adaptogens will work on the adrenal system, and more globally on the immune and endocrine systems.

ESSENTIAL

You should never use herbs to tax your adrenal gland system and continue to overstimulate the HPA axis. You want to use them to help you restore health to that area of the body, by helping you slow down and feel nourished. The only way you will get "more energy" for the long term is to use the plants wisely and not abuse them.

Here are some herbs that treat all stages of adrenal fatigue:

- Eleuthero (*Eleutherococcus senticosus*) is a great herb to promote mental clarity and improve emotional resilience when times are stressful. This herb is mildly energizing, so plan to use it when your cortisol levels are lower. It also helps with sleeplessness and supports the immune system. Warming.
- American ginseng (*Panax quinquefolius*) is a wonderful herb for promoting balance in the adrenal system without being overly energizing (it is less stimulating than Asian ginseng). It helps with mental clarity and mental alertness as well as memory. Warming.
- Asian ginseng (*Panax ginseng*) is energizing and is often used more in older individuals when there is a need for supporting the aging process. Generally considered a tonic, it is helpful with sexual function/vitality and when sheer physical exhaustion is present. Warming/hot.
- Holy basil/tulsi (*Ocimum sanctum*) keeps the adrenals from overreacting to stress and promotes a more steady stress response. Considered to be supportive of overall health and keeping the mind sharp. Warming.
- Schisandra (*Schisandra chinensis*) helps to improve concentration and is believed to calm the heart and quiet the spirit. It energizes the body without being overstimulating, helps reduce sleeplessness, and supports the immune system. Warming.
- Ashwagandha (*Withania somnifera*) is a general adaptogen tonic, used to help improve sexual function/stamina and promote a calm and restful sleep. It can be both stimulating and relaxing, depending on your constitution and what your body needs. Warming.
- Licorice (*Glycyrrhiza glabra*) is a nice herb if you need more cortisol in your body. It is wonderful for MSS3 and sometimes used preventatively in MSS1. It helps support the immune system, and can be used for allergies. Neutral to warming. This herb contains glycyrrhizic acid, which has been show to increase blood pressure in susceptible individuals. Long-term use is not warranted unless under the care of a practitioner with herbal medicine knowledge. There are also deglycyrrhizated forms of licorice in the marketplace. If you are currently on medications, please consult your qualified healthcare practitioner before using.
- Rhodiola (*Rhodiola rosea*) is great for helping the mind and brain better evaluate, analyze, and carry out a plan. It helps to support the heart after

stressful events and strengthens the immune system. Smaller doses are more stimulating, whereas larger doses are more sedating. Cooling and drying.

- Reishi mushroom (*Ganoderma lucidum*) is a great adaptogen that also supports the immune system and inflammatory response. It calms and strengthens the nervous system, and is considered a general tonic for overall health. At one point, this mushroom was only given to emperors, because it was just that special (and rare). Neutral to warming.
- Gotu kola (*Centella asiatica*) is a wonderful herb with a long tradition of use in Asian countries. It is used to promote wound healing, improve mental alertness, combat depression, and improve physical stamina. This herb has been used traditionally by yogis in India to help improve meditative practices. Cooling.

ALERT

You will need to do your homework and research herbs to understand what herb is best for you given your current medical health. You need to understand what contraindications may exist for an herb you decide to use, especially if you are on other natural therapies and/or pharmaceuticals. Please use multiple resources if you are planning to add an herbal remedy to your treatment plan and you are on pharmaceuticals.

Nervines

Nervines are a category of herbs that work to calm down and support the nervous system. Nervines are amazing medicine often used in conjunction with herbal adaptogens, since the nervous system is the main control for telling the HPA axis when to react to a stressor. Generally, you want to find a nervine that supports any other weakened systems in the body in addition to the adrenals. Following is a list of nervines that are helpful for both adrenal gland health and other systems you may have symptoms in (or are predisposed to having symptoms in).

- Chamomile (*Matricaria recutita*) is helpful when there is any sort of digestive system issue. It is antispasmodic, helping with headaches and muscle tension as well. Drying.
- Oat (*Avena sativa*) is a wonderful nervine that is gentle and nutritive to the body. It will help you feel more grounded in your body without sedation, and reduces fatigue when used as a daily herb. Moistening.
- Catnip (*Nepeta cataria*) is a mellow herb that is great for nervous headaches and is a gentle carminative (gas reliever). Cooling and drying.
- Lemon balm (*Melissa officinalis*) is a great tonic for the nervous system that is also helpful if immune support is needed, specifically viral immune support. Mildly warm.
- Skullcap (*Scutellaria lateriflora*) is great for when you have a lot of mental anxiety, including thoughts that go around in your head or the inability to let go of thoughts in order to rest or sleep. This herb is also mildly antispasmodic, helping to relieve muscle tension. Cooling.
- Lavender (*Lavandula angustifolia*) is a gentle nervine that helps reduce anxiety in the mind and often felt in the body. Helps to uplift the spirit and can promote a calm state for sleep. Cool, drying.
- Wood betony (*Stachys officinalis*) and hyssop (*Hyssopus officinalis*) are wonderful herbs to reduce inflammation by calming down an aberrant nervous system. Wood betony is great for reducing muscle tension, especially of the upper back, and hyssop is a gentle carminative. Drying.
- California poppy (*Eschscholzia californica*) is great if you really feel your stress response in your body and you have a lot of restlessness and pain. It can also help promote a deeper state of sleep. Cooling.
- Passionflower (*Passiflora incarnata*) is an extremely bitter nervine that is also wonderful for sleep issues and a restless mind. It helps improve digestive system function, especially when there is a slow or sluggish manner to it. Cooling.
- Valerian (*Valeriana officinalis*) is great when the primary goal is rest and deep sleep. Valerian is a fairly strong herb and has been known to cause stimulation in some people. Mildly warming.
- Kava (*Piper methysticum*) is a good nervine for those in hyperadrenia who may have sleep issues. It also treats headaches and muscle inflammation/spasms. It can be quite warming, though, so if you already experience hot flashes, it may not be the best herb for you.

Hormonal Agents for Adrenal Gland Health

Pregnenolone and DHEA (dehydroepiandrosterone) are considered non-glandular hormonal agents. Pregnenolone is the "rate-limiting step" from cholesterol to all steroid hormones, meaning that if you don't have enough, you won't produce cholesterol or cholesterol hormones. Remember that cholesterol is the building block for your adrenal hormones and your sex hormones. Without enough pregnenolone, the body will be fighting over whether to make adrenal hormones or sex hormones, and there are many in each category. Proper quantities of pregnenolone help the body have enough starting material to successfully make adequate hormone levels all around.

DHEA is a steroid hormone farther down the path to sex hormones. DHEA is sort of cortisol's balancer. There is about three to four times as much DHEA pumped out daily than there is cortisol. DHEA is responsible for creating androgens, including testosterone, and also supports estrogen production including three unique forms of estrogen, as well as hormone metabolites in each pathway.

Pregnenolone

Pregnenolone can be bought as a supplement. Either the sublingual (under the tongue) or the oral form is fine. You will need to take less of the sublingual one, because it absorbs into the bloodstream much faster when taken under the tongue—there is no "first pass" metabolism by the liver as there is with everything that is digested and absorbed in the small intestine.

Pregnenolone will mostly work to support the adrenal pathways to improve daytime wakefulness, which of course over time and with a comprehensive treatment plan will rebalance daytime energy levels and night-time sleep quality.

You may find that starting as low as 10mg is helpful for you. Some individuals need upwards of 50–100mg depending on the form (sublingual or oral), lab results, and severity of adrenal fatigue. At the higher dose most people generally only require 3–6 months of treatment. A tapering down is always the best with hormonally active supplements.

DHEA (Dehydroepiandrosterone)

DHEA is often used when lab values are low, and as a midline therapy when nutrients and herbs, as well as diet and lifestyle, are just not enough to give the adrenal glands what they need to heal. The dose is smaller, around 5–20mg.

You would start with 5mg daily for the course of a week, continually adding 5mg each week until you find your unique dose. Common side effects can be anxiety, irritability, facial hair, and acne; think of androgens and testosterone. If you reach this level, then you need to back down by 5mg and stay at this level for the duration of treatment. There is also 7-keto DHEA, which tends not to produce side effects as strongly as DHEA, but may be less effective. Once this has been used for the desired period of time (3–9 months), it should be tapered down.

Glandular Extract and Cortisone for Adrenal Gland Health

Glandular extract and cortisone can be very effective shorter-term therapies for those with severe adrenal fatigue. Both of these therapies tend to rest and then jump-start the adrenal glands in patients with hypoadrenia. Generally these therapies are used for 3–9 months, depending on the individual. They are not the only therapies used during this stage, nor do they have to be the first line used during this stage, but they are extremely effective for those who have tried other natural therapies without much success or who have been through a shock that has completely paralyzed the adrenal gland system.

You must be diligent when buying glandular extract (adrenal gland, pituitary, and hypothalamus from animal sources), as you want these therapies to be from clean sources. This means the animals were raised in their natural environment without the use of hormones and antibiotics, and preferably on an organic diet. You won't find the products themselves organic, but make sure the company uses quality animal adrenal gland. Please know that these organs are considered "waste" products, so animals are never slaughtered for them; rather these organs are used from animals already being raised for meat and dairy. If you consume animal, it is actually a great way to add more sustainability into animal practices, as the organs are not going to waste.

For cortisone, you will need a prescription for hydrocortisone, and your healthcare practitioner will decide the right dose for you. When coming off of both glandular and hydrocortisone, you will go through a tapering-down schedule. This is what will allow the body to come from an adrenal gland rest phase to a period where the adrenal gland begins to carry the workload of the stress response from a healed state. The additional therapies including vitamins, minerals, herbs, diet, and lifestyle changes you have made will provide the adrenals with the support they require during this transition. Eventually the herbs and nutrients can be tapered off, as the "basics" are able to maintain overall health.

Homeopathy for Adrenal Gland Health

Homeopathic remedies can be extremely invaluable for stimulating healing by the body. This is what is referred to as stimulating and supporting the vis. The vis is similar to what traditional Chinese and Japanese medicine refer to as chi or qi, the energy or life force of the body. This energy is what keeps you alive.

In natural Western medicine practices, supporting the vis, which can be done with homeopathy, allows for healing on a much gentler and individual basis. You can use homeopathy as a constitutional treatment, which means the remedy fits you as a person, or as an acute remedy, which means the treatment is more condition specific. Both have their place. You can also find some of the glandular hormones above in homeopathic dilation, which may be a preferred way of using these if you are sensitive to hormones, or don't necessarily desire consuming the whole glandular extract. Homeopathic remedies are prepared by dilution and succussion (shaking), a process that allows for the energy of the material being used to be potentiated. Homeopathic remedies are extremely effective when the right constitutional one is found.

Other Common Symptoms and Treatment

Beyond healing the adrenals, there are common symptoms that present with adrenal fatigue. For instance, cardiovascular disease including dyslipidemia and high blood pressure are fairly common complaints coinciding with adrenal fatigue, because the stress response is continually elevated and the cortisol output increases blood pressure, causes more oxidative stress, and damages the blood vessels.

Digestive complaints are also more common, as the adrenal glands and the stress response tend to cause a decrease in gastric function, causing you to not properly break down your food, potentially experience disturbances such as reflux, constipation, or diarrhea, and not absorb key nutrients, even when the diet is healthy.

Thyroid issues are common with adrenal fatigue, and many people who suffer with thyroid issues do not support their adrenal system properly. In order for the thyroid to heal, the adrenals must be healed, as the thyroid relies on the adrenals being healthy. Many individuals with thyroid disease not only aren't getting adrenal support, but most likely don't know it is probably an autoimmune condition (75 percent of Americans who have hypothyroidism actually have Hashimoto's thyroiditis). Being given only thyroid hormone does nothing for healing the autoimmunity or supporting the adrenal glands, or restoring health to the thyroid itself.

Additional Supplements to Consider

Omega-3 fats are often vital in helping reduce inflammation in the body, and promote long-term health in the cardiovascular system. You can get adequate amounts of omega-3 fats if you eat wild-caught fish a few times a week, as well as raw nuts and seeds rich in omega-3s, including walnut, pumpkin, and chia. You can also get a better profile of omega-3 fats from grass-fed red meats.

When looking to supplements, make sure to get oil from salmon or cod liver. Consuming supplements with fish oil from smaller fish (e.g., sardine and anchovies) is adding to the unsustainable harvesting of these small fish for fishmeal, as the oil is a leftover by-product. Using the oil is of course great, because it is not wasted, but the fishmeal industry needs to be re-evaluated for sustainability (please look at the fishmeal industry in Peru for more information on the deleterious health effects). The recommended dose is 1000–3000mg combined EPA (eicosapentaenoic acid) and DHA (docosahexaenoic acid).

L-carnitine can be a very helpful supplement for those with cardiovascular disease as well as mitochondrial dysfunction. L-carnitine helps to bring fats into the mitochondria for fuel burning, and therefore can aid in muscle energy needs. It supports healthy nitric oxide levels, which increases healthy relaxation in the blood vessels and reduces arrhythmias, symptoms of angina, and all-cause mortality. The proper dose is 2–3gms.

Coenzyme Q10 (CoQ10), otherwise known as ubiquinone or ubiquinol in the reduced form, is used by every cell in the body to produce energy in the mitochondria. This nutrient is depleted if you are taking statins, a cholesterol-lowering medication, and it is vital to your health and energy levels. If you are struggling with dyslipidemia or energy and brain fatigue, CoQ10 may be the right supplement for you. Generally you will take 100mg of ubiquinol or 100–200mg ubiquinone, as your body will have to convert the latter and some does not necessarily get converted, so a higher dose may be needed.

D-ribose can help jump-start the body's energy by contributing to the generation of ATP. D-ribose is a sugar, but it is not like glucose or fructose; it is different and the body will phosphorylate it, by adding a phosphate group to it, to create more ATP, which is great for you if you have severely low energy, often the case in MSS3.

Phosphatidylserine has been shown to improve parameters of memory and focus. It is also considered useful in adrenal fatigue as it supports the breakdown of cortisol, and thus may help to alleviate high levels of cortisol at specific times of the day. A 2014 study in the *Journal of Human Nutrition and Dietetics* showed that phosphatidylserine was helpful for children with ADHD by significantly improving inattention, short-term auditory memory, and impulsivity. In a 2010 study in the *Journal of Clinical Interventions in Aging*, phosphatidylserine was shown to improve subjective memory complaints along with omega-3 supplements. Phosphatidylerine is generally dosed at 100mg to start. Using it about 1 hour before higher cortisol times during the day or before bed is recommended.

FACT

Paying attention to what other symptoms you have in your body and how they respond to your adrenal gland treatment will tell you how much of your adrenal dysfunction was affecting this area of your body. As your adrenal glands and HPA axis heal and you remove nutritional therapies that did the job, you will be able to see which symptoms stay healed and which may need additional support. This is just part of the road to full recovery and optimal wellness.

Whether you decide to use a supplement or you get your probiotics from eating fermented and cultured foods daily, one thing is for sure, you need to consume probiotics for optimal health. They will support a healthy digestive system and immune system (remember that 70 percent of your immune system lives in your gut). Probiotics signal neurotransmitters, which communicate with your brain and central nervous system. They also turn your DNA on and off. Generally a 25 billion 8–12 multi strain is the best. You want supplements that list both the genus (Lactobacillus) and species (acidophilus), and preferably the strain type (DDS-1) as well.

Example Treatment Protocols for MSS1–MSS3

By now you are probably swimming with information, and you get to put it all together to come up with the best treatment plan for yourself. In order to help you do this, there are three "treatment examples" you should refer to when trying to create your own individual treatment plan. You will want to use the **10-Step Plan** as the map, and then look to the treatment examples of MSS1, MSS2, and MSS3 to help you fill in steps 7–10 of the **10-Step Plan**, specifically.

QUESTION

Are supplements the only thing to use to heal adrenal fatigue?
Absolutely not. In fact, if you try to heal your adrenal glands and HPA axis with nutritional therapies alone, you are doing yourself a disservice. For one thing, your supplements will work much better if you also do all the dietary and lifestyle recommendations. And second, when you pull the supplements away, the majority of symptoms may come back. Do yourself a favor and get started on the right foot.

MSS1 Example Treatment

Nutritional therapies include 500mg vitamin C two times a day with a food. B-complex: 1 with breakfast and 1 with lunch. No coffee in the morning; instead, organic green tea. Holy basil tea for an afternoon pick-me-up.

Ashwagandha 500mg and magnesium 250mg, 1 hour prior to bed to promote a restful sleep (if sleep issues are present). You should have a 25B multi-strain probiotic with dinner each night and 15mg of zinc at the beginning of each meal taken three times a day (if digestive sluggishness is present). Chamomile and catnip tea as needed to help with bloating and gas.

MSS2 Example Treatment

Nutritional therapies include vitamin B_5, 100mg two times a day, in the morning and afternoon. Take vitamin B_6 50mg daily at 2 P.M., along with a trace mineral complex and an adrenal product with rhodiola, passionflower, ashwagandha, holy basil, and L-theanine (all calming down an overstimulated mind and body). No coffee; instead drink an oat, hyssop, and lemon balm tea every morning. Take CoQ10 to treat high blood pressure at 100mg reduced form, as well as 2gm L-carnitine to prevent cardiovascular disease (family history), and omega-3 fats 2000mg daily at breakfast. Take probiotic 25B multistrain with dinner. Take 10mg DHEA mid-morning and mid-afternoon, if DHEA lab levels came back low.

Take 5000IU vitamin A (retinyl palmitate) to support healthy production of secretory IgA (if you are susceptible to getting ill). Take 100mg phosphatidylserine at night about 1 hour prior to bed, as well as 250mg magnesium, if nighttime cortisol is elevated and causing insomnia. Take a sleepy-time tincture if needed. If you wake in the middle of the night and can't fall back asleep, take valerian, California poppy, passionflower, lavender, skullcap, and oats. Take 2 droppersful in a small amount of water. This can be repeated as needed until rest is achieved, up to 3 to 4 doses.

MSS3 Example Treatment

Nutritional therapies include 25mg sublingual pregnenolone morning and early afternoon. Try taking an herbal tincture of American ginseng, eleuthero, ashwagandha, schisandra, and ginger mid-morning and mid-afternoon, 2 droppersful in a small amount of water. Licorice solid extract: ½ teaspoon in the morning before breakfast and ½ teaspoon before lunch. Take D-ribose 5gm daily in water to help boost energy levels, during lowest energy time for you. Probiotic 25B multistrain taken with dinner. Homeopathic adrenal glandular extract, (surreninum) 4CH (homeopathic dilution):

take 1 dose daily (3–4 pellets), allowed to dissolve under the tongue in the morning upon waking, 20 minutes away from food and beverage. Vitamin B_5: 250mg; vitamin B6: 100mg; vitamin B_3: 75mg divided over 2 doses daily with food (preferably breakfast and lunch). Vitamin B_{12} and methylfolate: 1000mcg and 800mcg lozenge allowed to dissolve under the tongue each morning. Oat and holy basil tea every afternoon. Take 300mg magnesium in mid-morning and before bed every day.

The 10-Step Plan to Healing Adrenal Fatigue

The purpose of this book is to help you put together the pieces to create a customized treatment plan using all of the basic foundations of health, as well as nutritional therapies, to fill in the gaps and accelerate the healing process. This will set you in motion on the path of optimal health.

The 10-Step Plan will allow you to lay out the road map to healing your adrenal glands. All you need to do is fill in the information from the various treatment sections including dietary recommendations to restore health to the adrenals, lifestyle recommendations to flip your disease-promoting habits into health-promoting habits, and appropriate nutritional therapies. You have the map; now just plug in the pieces specific to what stage of adrenal fatigue you fall into.

The pre-step to the 10-Step Plan is to understand what stage of adrenal fatigue you are in, based on appropriate lab work, completing the adrenal gland assessment questionnaire, and performing the home tests (if desired).

Putting It All Together

1. **Begin by assessing your diet.** No matter how many supplements you use, if your diet does not support adrenal health, your supplements won't be as effective as they should be and you won't be able to go off of them without your symptoms coming back. Your diet may adapt as you heal your adrenals, and that is fine. Start with the recommendations for what stage of adrenal fatigue you are in, to be sure to eat what supports your health.

2. **Get your (quality) sleep.** In order for your adrenal rhythm to come back into balance, whether it is in hyperadrenia or hypoadrenia, you will need to make sure your sleep-wake cycle is in balance. If your sleep cycle is disrupted, this is an absolute must in your map.

3. **Mindfulness-based practices.** Your mind is one extremely powerful vehicle for positive change. In order to change your external world, you must change your internal world. No matter who you are or what health struggle you encounter, you must use mindfulness-based practices including yoga, meditation, earthing, and deep breathing to bring a deeper sense of awareness, connection, and purpose to your daily life. This in itself is quite healing.

4. **Exercise, movement, and sweating.** You must exercise. Humans are not meant to live sedentary lifestyles. Your life expectancy actually decreases the more hours you sit during your life. Be sure to do the right type of exercise for your stage of adrenal fatigue, and please get outside for some fresh air. Maybe you will do both of those activities together!

5. **Fresh air and deep breathing.** Your lungs are amazing organs. They are able to take in oxygen and transfer it to your blood for your body to have all the oxygen it needs to feed the mitochondria and generate ATP. The lungs also help you to connect to Mother Nature and process your grief, as the lungs are where grief is stored in the body, according to such healing arts as traditional Chinese medicine. Deep breathing helps reduce anxiety, gives you stable energy to heal the adrenals, and allows you to slow down in life.

6. **Self-care through the ages.** Do you ever notice how children retreat when they need alone time? You need to create your own alone time. Connecting with yourself and giving yourself space from others is vital to health and longevity. Yes, humans are communal beings, but even the most outgoing individual still needs some alone time to check in and make sure she is connecting with her spiritual or religious beliefs. Having a connection to something greater than yourself gives you meaning and purpose, which of course reduces stress and heals the adrenal glands.

7. **Vitamins and minerals.** This is where you take what stage you are in, combined with what symptoms you experience, and put those together to find the best natural vitamins and minerals to support your recovery.

Refer back to the nutrients and why they are used beginning in Chapter 10. Decide which are good for you by looking at each MSS1–MSS3 rating.

8. **Herbs and other adrenal support.** Similar to vitamins and minerals, refer back to the other treatments provided and decide whether they would be applicable to your current stage of adrenal fatigue and symptom picture.

9. **Supporting detoxification pathways.** This is crucial to overall health and longevity. Your body naturally detoxifies on a daily basis and you want to support that by some of the health-promoting habits: drinking water, exercising, being in the sun, getting fresh air, deep breathing, and sweating. Start by adding one new support in each month, or even add in two a month. You will be seeing your health improve over time, and these habits will stick with you to keep you healthy long after you have healed your adrenal fatigue.

10. **Treating other symptoms.** Of course, if you suffer from systemic symptoms you will want to focus on healing those as well. You will see that a thorough adrenal gland treatment will help. You may also need additional therapies to heal symptoms, depending on severity and duration as well as what you have been using to treat them up until now. You have information on some of the most common "other symptoms" that individuals with adrenal fatigue present with and what you should use to treat these symptoms, so start there and adapt as you heal.

Now you know what you need to do to treat, heal, and cure your adrenal fatigue. You deserve only the best in your health. Here is to a forward path in recovery as you learn more about yourself and stretch and grow every day. Life is a journey to be lived, so make sure each day you are really living life to the fullest. When you are healing, remember the road is often two steps forward and one step back. Don't get discouraged; just continue forward. You ought to have the best health you can have; you just need to know how to get it and what to do to maintain it. Here's to health and vitality!

CHAPTER 12

Smoothies

A Berry Great Morning

This smoothie is packed with antioxidants, powerful phytochemicals, and protein that will get you moving and keep you moving!

INGREDIENTS | YIELDS 1 QUART

2 cups mixed baby greens
1 pint raspberries
1 pint blueberries
½ avocado
1 cup milk (organic or alternative milk)

1. Combine greens, berries, and avocado and blend thoroughly.

2. While blending, add milk slowly until desired texture is achieved.

PER 1 CUP SERVING: Calories: 184 | Fat: 7 g | Protein: 4 g | Sodium: 33 mg | Fiber: 9 g | Carbohydrates: 29 g | Sugar: 17 g | GI: Moderate

Blueberries and Raspberries for a Healthy Life

Combining raspberries and blueberries in the same smoothie gives your immune system a boost. The vitamins and phytochemicals that burst from these berries and make their skin the vibrant red and purple are what also help fight off the carcinogens and provide you with antioxidants to keep you feeling your best.

Great Grapefruit

The grapefruit and cucumber combine in this smoothie to offer a refreshing zing to your morning. This smoothie's vitamins and nutrients will wake you up and keep you feeling fresh throughout the day!

INGREDIENTS | YIELDS 1 QUART

1 cup baby greens
2 grapefruits, peeled
1 cucumber, peeled and sliced
¼ cup purified water

1. Combine greens, grapefruit, and cucumber with half of the water and blend.

2. Add remaining water slowly while blending until desired consistency is reached.

PER 1 CUP SERVING: Calories: 59 | Fat: 0 g | Protein: 1 g | Sodium: 3 mg | Fiber: 2 g | Carbohydrates: 14 g | Sugar: 6 g | GI: Low

Luscious Lemon-Lime

The tartness of lemons and limes is balanced with crisp romaine and sweet stevia, with no calories. The kefir gives this smoothie a creamy texture with protein and essential vitamins. Drinking this smoothie will help you feel awake and refreshed.

INGREDIENTS | YIELDS 2 CUPS

1 cup romaine lettuce
2 lemons, peeled
2 limes, peeled
½ cup kefir
1 dropperful of liquid stevia

1. Combine romaine, lemons, limes, and kefir and blend until thoroughly combined.

2. Add stevia slowly while blending, stopping periodically to taste, until desired sweetness and texture are achieved.

PER 1 CUP SERVING: Calories: 81 | Fat: 2 g | Protein: 3 g | Sodium: 35 mg | Fiber: 4 g | Carbohydrates: 17 g | Sugar: 6 g | GI: Low

Balance Your Body

Not only do lemons and limes have the acidity and tang to make you pucker up, but they are incredibly healthy, too. Those same small, sour fruits that can bring a tear to your eye actually promote a balanced alkaline level in your body.

Calming Cucumber

The light taste of cucumber and powerfully fragrant mint combine with deep green romaine in this delightfully smooth and refreshing smoothie. Not only can this be a great start to your day, but it can also be a great way to unwind at the end of it.

INGREDIENTS | YIELDS 3–4 CUPS

1 cup romaine lettuce
2 cucumbers, peeled
¼ cup mint, chopped
1 cup purified water, divided

1. Place romaine, cucumbers, mint, and ½ cup water in a blender and combine thoroughly.

2. Add remaining water while blending until desired texture is achieved.

PER 1 CUP SERVING: Calories: 24 | Fat: 0 g | Protein: 1 g | Sodium: 9 mg | Fiber: 2 g | Carbohydrates: 4 g | Sugar: 3 g | GI: Very low

The Slump Bumper

With the energizing effects of natural sugars (fructose) found in sweet fruits and vegetables, there's no comparison to energy drinks or junk foods that give you quick, but short-lived, energy.

INGREDIENTS | YIELDS 4 CUPS

1 cup spinach
2 pears, cored and peeled
1 cup cherries, pitted
½ avocado
2 cups almond milk, divided

Benefits of Cherries

Packed with an assortment of vitamins and minerals, an obvious sign from their intense red color, cherries help mental functions such as memory. Cherries also improve energy, and promote focus and attention.

1. Place spinach, pears, cherries, avocado, and 1 cup of almond milk in a blender and blend until thoroughly combined.

2. Add remaining cup of almond milk while blending until desired texture is achieved.

PER 1 CUP SERVING: Calories: 128 | Fat: 5 g | Protein: 2 g | Sodium: 98 mg | Fiber: 8 g | Carbohydrates: 22 g | Sugar: 13 g | GI: Moderate

Peachy Berry

If you love peaches and berries, combining them with the baby greens in this smoothie delivers sweet tastes with vitamins and nutrients.

INGREDIENTS | YIELDS 3 CUPS

1 cup baby greens
2 peaches, pitted and peeled
1 cup strawberries
½ cup coconut milk
½ tablespoon fresh ginger, sliced or grated

1. Add all ingredients to a blender and blend until thoroughly combined.

2. Add water, if necessary, while blending if smoothie is too thick.

PER 1 CUP SERVING: Calories: 51 | Fat: 1 g | Protein: 2 g | Sodium: 18 mg | Fiber: 4 g | Carbohydrates: 11 g | Sugar: 8 g | GI: Low

Minty Bliss

The ingredients here blend together to create a sweet treat with a creamy texture; this smoothie may be satisfying enough to bump your favorite ice cream out of its number one spot!

INGREDIENTS | YIELDS 3 CUPS

1 cup iceberg lettuce
¼ cup whole mint leaves
1 pint raspberries
1 cup almond milk
½ cup Greek-style yogurt

1. Place the lettuce, mint, raspberries, and almond milk in a blender and blend until thoroughly combined.

2. Add yogurt while blending until desired texture is achieved.

PER 1 CUP SERVING: Calories: 86 | Fat: 1 g | Protein: 5 g | Sodium: 54 mg | Fiber: 6 g | Carbohydrates: 16 g | Sugar: 6 g | GI: Low

Cleansing Cranberry

If you're looking for a sweet and tangy treat, this smoothie is for you. The combination of cranberries, cucumber, lemon, and ginger give this smoothie the power to cleanse your body while delivering a taste sensation.

INGREDIENTS | YIELDS 4–6 CUPS

1 cup watercress
2 pints cranberries
2 cucumbers, peeled
½ lemon, peeled
1 (½") piece fresh ginger, peeled
2 cups purified water, divided

1. Place watercress, cranberries, cucumbers, lemon, ginger, and 1 cup of purified water in a blender and blend until thoroughly combined.

2. Add the remaining 1 cup of water while blending, as needed, until desired texture is achieved.

PER 1 CUP SERVING: Calories: 41 | Fat: 0 g | Protein: 1 g | Sodium: 7 mg | Fiber: 4 g | Carbohydrates: 10 g | Sugar: 5 g | GI: Very low

Blueberry Antioxidant Smoothie

Blueberries contain one of the highest antioxidant levels found in fruit. This smoothie is refreshing as it fights free-radical oxidation in your body.

INGREDIENTS | SERVES 1

1 cup frozen blueberries
½ avocado
1 cup vanilla-flavored almond milk
⅛ teaspoon ground nutmeg
4–6 ice cubes

Combine all the ingredients in a blender and purée until smooth.

PER SERVING: Calories: 329 | Fat: 17 g | Protein: 13 g | Sodium: 141 mg | Fiber: 11 g | Carbohydrates: 39 g | Sugar: 5 g | GI: Low

Almond Joy Smoothie

This chocolate-and-coconut smoothie is a real treat when you are craving something sweet.

INGREDIENTS | SERVES 2

1 cup coconut milk
½ cup cacao nibs
3 tablespoons raw honey
½ teaspoon ground cinnamon
¼ teaspoon ground nutmeg
4–6 ice cubes

Combine all the ingredients in a blender and purée until smooth.

PER SERVING: Calories: 395 | Fat: 28 g | Protein: 2.5 g | Sodium: 16 mg | Fiber: 0 g | Carbohydrates: 39.5 g | Sugar: 7.5 g | GI: Moderate

CHAPTER 13

Juices

Spicy Cucumber

Cucumbers are rich in chlorophyll and silica.
They are a natural diuretic and benefit digestion.

INGREDIENTS | YIELDS 1 CUP

1 cucumber
1 clove garlic, peeled
2 green onions, trimmed
½ jalapeño pepper
2 small key limes or Mexican limes

1. Process the ingredients in any order through a masticating juicer according to the manufacturer's directions.

2. Stir to mix the juice and serve over ice.

PER SERVING: Calories: 98 | Fat: 1 g | Protein: 3.5 g | Sodium: 12 mg | Carbohydrates: 27 g | Sugar: 9 g | GI: Low

Vegetable Super Juice

Add a generous dash of hot sauce to this juice for extra zip!
It's great on the rocks for a fast summer lunch.

INGREDIENTS | YIELDS 1½ CUPS

1 whole cucumber
6 leaves romaine lettuce
4 stalks celery, including leaves
2 cups fresh spinach
½ cup alfalfa sprouts
½ cup fresh parsley

Sandy Spinach?

Spinach grows best in sandy soils, but can be tough to really rinse well. Rather than rinsing spinach through a colander, place it in a deep bowl or kettle and cover it with water. Gently toss to allow any sand or grit to fall to the bottom and lift the greens out.

1. Cut the cucumber into pieces and process through your juicer according to the manufacturer's directions.

2. Wrap the lettuce leaves around the celery stalks and add to the feeding tube.

3. Add the spinach, sprouts, and parsley in any order you desire.

4. Mix the juice thoroughly before serving.

PER SERVING: Calories: 127 | Fat: 1.5 g | Protein: 8 g | Sodium: 212 mg | Carbohydrates: 25 g | Sugar: 10 g | GI: Low

The Energizer

Need a jolt? This concoction will perk you up and keep you on your toes.

INGREDIENTS | YIELDS 2 CUPS

2 apples, cored
½ cucumber
¼ bulb fennel
3 stalks celery, including leaves
½ lemon, peeled
1 (¼") piece fresh ginger
½ cup kale
½ cup spinach
6 leaves romaine lettuce

1. Slice the apples and process through the feed tube of an electronic juicer according to the manufacturer's directions.

2. Follow with pieces of cucumber and fennel.

3. Add the celery, followed by the lemon and the ginger.

4. Lightly tear the remaining greens into pieces and process.

5. Mix the juice thoroughly before serving. Serve over ice if desired.

PER SERVING: Calories: 277 | Fat: 1.8 g | Protein: 7.5 g | Sodium: 170 mg | Carbohydrates: 67 g | Sugar: 40 g | GI: Moderate

Mean Green Machine

Got a full day ahead? This one will make sure you get through it with energy to spare.

INGREDIENTS | YIELDS 2½ CUPS

1 cup fresh pineapple, peeled and chopped
1 medium Granny Smith apple, cored
2 cups baby spinach leaves
¼ cup parsley
2 tablespoons mint leaves
½ pink grapefruit, peeled and seeded
1 cup coconut water

1. Process the pineapple chunks in an electronic juicer according to the manufacturer's directions.

2. Slice the apple and add pieces to the juicer, maintaining the juicer speed.

3. Wash the spinach, parsley, and mint. Add to the juicer.

4. Add the grapefruit segments.

5. Whisk the juice together with the coconut water until well blended. Chill or serve immediately over ice.

PER SERVING: Calories: 246 | Fat: 1 g | Protein: 5 g | Sodium: 70 mg | Carbohydrates: 61 g | Sugar: 44 g | GI: Moderate

Glamorous Greens

Watercress and arugula both help activate enzymes in the liver, while acting as natural diuretics. Plus, they contribute a lively, peppery flavor that makes this one taste like it's fresh from the spa!

INGREDIENTS | YIELDS 1½ CUPS

½ bunch spinach, about 2 cups
1 cup watercress
1 cup arugula
1 medium apple, cored
½ lemon, peeled
2 stalks celery, with leaves
1 (½") piece fresh ginger

Juicing Greens

To make juicing green leafy vegetables such as lettuce and spinach easier, roll the greens into balls before adding to the juicer.

1. Rinse the spinach, watercress, and arugula well to ensure greens are free of grit.

2. Process the apple through an electronic juicer according to the manufacturer's directions.

3. Add the lemon and celery stalks.

4. Add the greens and ginger in any order.

5. Whisk the juice to combine and serve well-chilled or over ice.

PER SERVING: Calories: 148 | Fat: 1 g | Protein: 7.5 g | Sodium: 218 mg | Carbohydrates: 33 g | Sugar: 19 g | GI: Moderate

Super Cocktail

Vary the greens in this recipe according to your tastes and the season. It's guaranteed to fill you up, without filling you out! If you are hypothyroid, it is best not to consume raw brassicas including cabbage and kale, so replace those with romaine and arugula.

INGREDIENTS | YIELDS 2 CUPS
(2 SERVINGS)

2 stalks celery, including leaves
½ cucumber
¼ head green cabbage
2 stalks bok choy
½ medium apple, cored
½ lemon, peeled
1 (½") piece fresh ginger
½ cup parsley
5 kale or collard leaves
1 cup spinach

1. Process the celery and cucumber through a masticating juicer according to the manufacturer's directions.

2. Cut the cabbage into chunks and add to the juicer, followed by the bok choy, apple, and lemon.

3. Add the ginger and parsley.

4. Add the kale or collards, and the spinach.

5. Serve alone or over ice.

PER SERVING: Calories: 214 | Fat: 2 g | Protein: 11 g | Sodium: 188 mg | Carbohydrates: 47 g | Sugar: 17 g | GI: Moderate

A Hidden Clove

*The sweetness of the carrots will offset the strong taste of garlic,
and the dill adds a touch of green. This juice is great for reducing water retention.*

INGREDIENTS | YIELDS 1 CUP

4 carrots, peeled
2 garlic cloves, peeled
1 sprig baby dill

1. Process carrots and garlic through a masticating juicer according to the manufacturer's directions.

2. Garnish juice with baby dill.

PER SERVING: Calories: 91 | Fat: 0.5 g | Protein: 2 g | Sodium: 139 mg | Carbohydrates: 21 g | Sugar: 9 g | GI: Low

Beet Surprise

*Filling and flavorful. The surprise is that the addition of mint
enhances the sweetness and flavor of this recipe.*

INGREDIENTS | YIELDS 1 CUP

2 small beets, trimmed, with greens
1 large Granny Smith apple, cored
¼ cup fresh mint

1. Process the beets and the apple through a masticating juicer according to the manufacturer's directions.

2. Add the mint.

3. Stir or shake the juice together with some ice and enjoy!

PER SERVING: Calories: 158 | Fat: 0.6 g | Protein: 4 g | Sodium: 136 mg | Carbohydrates: 38 g | Sugar: 26 g | GI: Moderate

Health Harvest Special

In late summer and early autumn, it's hard to come home from the farmers' market without feeling that you've just bought more than you could ever eat! Juicing is a great way to manage nature's bounty and take advantage of all the goodness the season provides.

INGREDIENTS | YIELDS 1½ CUPS

1 small beet, greens optional
6 carrots, trimmed
2 stalks celery, with leaves
1 cucumber
1 grapefruit, peeled
1 kiwi fruit, peeled or unpeeled
1 red or black plum, pitted
2 Bosch or Anjou pears, cored
2 apples, cored

1. Process the beet and carrots through a masticating juicer according to the manufacturer's directions.

2. Add the celery and cucumber.

3. Add the grapefruit sections, followed by the kiwi.

4. Add the plum and the pears, followed by the apple.

5. Whisk or shake the juice to combine and serve over ice, if desired.

PER SERVING: Calories: 634 | Fat: 2.5 g | Protein: 11 g | Sodium: 347 mg | Carbohydrates: 158 g | Sugar: 9.7 g | GI: Low

Cabbage and Carrot Creation

You may also substitute red cabbage in this recipe, but be aware that while red cabbage is slightly higher in nutrients than the white or green varieties, it does have a stronger flavor. If you are hypothyroid, raw cabbage is best avoided.

INGREDIENTS | YIELDS 1 CUP

8 ounces white or green cabbage, chopped
3 large carrots, trimmed

1. Process the cabbage and carrots through an electronic juicer according to the manufacturer's directions.

2. Whisk or shake the juice to combine the ingredients and serve over ice.

PER SERVING: Calories: 144 | Fat: 0.7 g | Protein: 4.8 g | Sodium: 189 mg | Carbohydrates: 33 g | Sugar: 17 g | GI: Moderate

Read the Directions . . .

Cabbage, because of its high fiber content, can be challenging to some juicers, so be sure to check the manufacturer's guidelines.

CHAPTER 14

Breakfast

Herbed Omelet with Vegetables

This omelet is a simple and healthy way to add an extra serving of vegetables to your day.

INGREDIENTS | SERVES 2

2 tablespoons water
2 cups sliced white mushrooms
3 tablespoons 2% milk, divided
2 tablespoons sour cream
Salt and pepper to taste
2 tablespoons chopped green onions
1 tablespoon chopped chives
¼ teaspoon dried tarragon
4 eggs

Use Coconut Milk Instead

If you prefer to make a dairy-free omelet, use full-fat coconut milk in place of the milk and sour cream listed. It will make the omelet creamy and delicious, and it doesn't taste like coconuts.

1. Heat a large skillet on medium-high heat and add 2 tablespoons of water. Add the mushrooms and sauté until they are soft and the liquid evaporates, about 3–4 minutes.

2. In a medium bowl, mix together 1 tablespoon of milk, sour cream, salt, and pepper. Whisk well and set aside.

3. In another medium bowl, mix the remaining 2 tablespoons of milk, green onion, chives, tarragon, and eggs; stir well.

4. Pour the egg mixture into a greased pan over medium-high heat; spread it evenly over the pan. Once the center is cooked, cover the egg with the mushrooms. Loosen the omelet with a spatula and fold it over.

5. Place the omelet on a plate to serve and top with the sour cream mixture.

PER SERVING: Calories: 164 | Fat: 9 g | Protein: 17 g | Sodium: 108 mg | Fiber: 0 g | Carbohydrates: 5 g | Sugar: 1 g | GI: Very low

Mini Quiche

These are a tasty treat for breakfast and can be made in bulk.

INGREDIENTS | SERVES 8

Olive oil, as needed

6 large eggs

6 slices bacon

1 tablespoon butter

½ cup chopped broccoli

½ cup sliced mushrooms

½ cup diced onions

½ cup diced organic red bell pepper

1. Preheat the oven to 325°F. Line a muffin tin with 8 foil muffin cups and brush cups with olive oil.

2. Whisk the eggs in a medium bowl and set them aside.

3. Cook the bacon in a medium frying pan over medium heat until crisp, drain on paper towels, and chop into ½" pieces.

4. Add butter to the bacon pan and sauté the remaining ingredients for 5 minutes.

5. Pour the eggs into foil cups, filling each two-thirds of the way.

6. Add the bacon and vegetables to each cup.

7. Bake 25 minutes or until golden brown.

PER SERVING: Calories: 131 | Fat: 10 g | Protein: 8 g | Sodium: 198 mg | Fiber: 0.5 g | Carbohydrates: 2 g | Sugar: 1 g | GI: Very low

Poached Eggs with Steamed Greens

Poached eggs are very quick to make, but you must watch them or they will overcook.
Time them exactly to get a perfect poached egg every time.

INGREDIENTS | SERVES 1

Water

1 teaspoon apple cider vinegar

2 large eggs

1 cup steamed organic kale, collard greens, or Swiss chard

1. Bring the water to a boil in a medium saucepan. Reduce the heat to medium-low so that the water is simmering.

2. Add the vinegar to the water.

3. Crack and carefully slide the eggs into the water.

4. Cook for exactly 3 minutes, and remove with a slotted spoon.

5. Plate the steamed kale, gently place eggs on top, and serve.

PER SERVING: Calories: 186 | Fat: 10 g | Protein: 14.5 g | Sodium: 156 mg | Fiber: 2.6 g | Carbohydrates: 4.6 g | Sugar: 1.6 g | GI: Very low

Paleo Breakfast Bowl

This breakfast is a bit more exciting than an ordinary breakfast.
Nitrate-free, uncured bacon is a real treat.

INGREDIENTS | SERVES 1

1 cup diced asparagus

½ cup diced bacon

2 large eggs

1. Add the asparagus to the skillet with bacon and cook until the asparagus is not quite tender, about 8–10 minutes. Remove to a small bowl.

2. In the same skillet, cook the eggs sunny-side up (do not flip) about 5 minutes. Be sure that the yolks are runny.

3. Place the cooked eggs on top of the bacon mixture.

4. Mix and serve.

PER SERVING: Calories: 321 | Fat: 28 g | Protein: 23 g | Sodium: 534 mg | Fiber: 3 g | Carbohydrates: 7.5 g | Sugar: 0 g | GI: Very low

Egg Muffins

These are great to make in advance and take with you.
They are also quite tasty with sliced avocado.

INGREDIENTS | SERVES 18

2 tablespoons olive oil
12 large eggs
2 medium zucchini
1 organic bell pepper, seeded and chopped
1 green onion
3 cups fresh organic spinach
1 cup cubed cooked ham

1. Preheat the oven to 350°F.

2. Grease two muffin pans with olive oil.

3. In a large bowl, whisk the eggs well.

4. In a food processor, process the zucchini, pepper, and green onion until finely chopped but not smooth.

5. Add the chopped vegetables to the eggs.

6. Finely chop the spinach in the food processor and add to the egg mixture.

7. Stir in the ham and mix well.

8. Fill the muffin pans halfway with the egg mixture.

9. Bake for 20–25 minutes or until the eggs are set in the middle.

PER SERVING: Calories: 75 | Fat: 5 g | Protein: 5 g | Sodium: 108 mg | Fiber: 0.5 g | Carbohydrates: 2 g | Sugar: 1 g | GI: Very low

Spinach, Egg, and Bacon Breakfast Salad

Salad isn't just for lunch and dinner anymore.
When you are following a low-GI plan, salads are round-the clock meals.

INGREDIENTS | SERVES 2

3 cups organic baby spinach leaves

4 large eggs, hard-boiled, peeled, and quartered

2 slices bacon, cooked and chopped

½ cup sliced cucumber

½ avocado, diced

½ organic apple, sliced

Juice of ½ lemon

1. Divide the spinach leaves on 2 plates and top each with 2 eggs and half the bacon.

2. Add cucumber, avocado, and apple slices to the top of the salads.

3. Squeeze fresh lemon juice over each salad. Serve immediately.

PER SERVING: Calories: 347 | Fat: 22 g | Protein: 20 g | Sodium: 334 mg | Fiber: 5 g | Carbohydrates: 16 g | Sugar: 2.5 g | GI: Low

Salmon Omelet

This omelet is full of omega-3 fatty acids. It is well seasoned and will surely become a breakfast staple.

INGREDIENTS | SERVES 2

2 tablespoons olive oil

¼ cup chopped green onions

1 cup trimmed and chopped asparagus

1 tablespoon chopped fresh dill

6 ounces salmon

6 large eggs, beaten

1. In a large skillet over medium heat, combine the olive oil, green onions, asparagus, and fresh dill. Sauté until the asparagus is soft, 5–10 minutes. Place in a bowl and set aside.

2. In the same skillet, sauté the salmon until flaky, about 10 minutes depending on the thickness of the steak. Place in a bowl and set aside.

3. Wipe out the skillet and cook the eggs on both sides until lightly browned, about 5 minutes each side.

4. Place the salmon mixture on half of the egg, fold over, and serve.

PER SERVING: Calories: 490 | Fat: 33 g | Protein: 40 g | Sodium: 332 mg | Fiber: 4 g | Carbohydrates: 9 g | Sugar: 1 g | GI: Very low

Slow Cooker Eggs Florentine

*Freshly ground black pepper goes well in this dish. You can use up to a teaspoon in the recipe.
If you prefer to season lightly to accommodate individual tastes,
be sure to have a pepper grinder at the table for those who want to add more.*

INGREDIENTS | SERVES 4

1 (8-ounce) package mushrooms

2 teaspoons olive oil

Butter, as needed

9 ounces (2 cups) grated Cheddar cheese, divided

1 (10-ounce) package organic frozen spinach, thawed

1 small onion, peeled and diced

6 large eggs

1 cup heavy cream

½ teaspoon Italian seasoning

½ teaspoon garlic powder

½ teaspoon freshly ground black pepper

Make It Dairy-Free

To make egg casseroles dairy-free, replace the cream with full-fat coconut milk. There are many dairy-free alternatives available for Cheddar cheese; one, in particular, sold by Daiya Foods, is available shredded and melts beautifully in dishes like this.

1. Clean the mushrooms by wiping with a damp towel. Trim and slice mushrooms. Place olive oil in a large skillet; heat over medium heat. Add mushrooms and cook until softened and all liquid has evaporated, about 10 minutes.

2. Grease a 4-quart slow cooker with butter. Spread 1 cup of the grated cheese over the bottom of the slow cooker.

3. Drain the spinach, squeezing out any excess moisture, and add it in a layer on top of the cheese. Next, add the sliced mushrooms in a layer and then top them with the onion.

4. In a medium bowl, beat the eggs, cream, Italian seasoning, garlic powder, and pepper. Pour the mixture over the layers in the slow cooker. Top with the remaining cup of cheese.

5. Cover and cook on high for 2 hours or until the eggs are set.

PER SERVING: Calories: 670 | Fat: 57.5 g | Protein: 30 g | Sodium: 712 mg | Fiber: 3 g | Carbohydrates: 11 g | Sugar: 3 g | GI: Low

Grain-Free, Egg-Free Pancakes

A common challenge with grain-free or low-glycemic gluten-free baking is figuring out how to make recipes without eggs. These pancakes use chia seeds as the binding ingredient instead.

INGREDIENTS | SERVES 4

2 tablespoons chia seeds

6 tablespoons warm water

1½ cups blanched almond flour

1 tablespoon arrowroot starch or tapioca starch

½ teaspoon sea salt

½ teaspoon baking soda

½ teaspoon ground cinnamon

¼ cup unsweetened organic applesauce or plain pumpkin purée

½ cup almond milk

1½ teaspoons vanilla extract

Pure maple syrup or honey

2 tablespoons butter or coconut oil

1. In a small bowl, whisk the chia seeds and warm water. Set aside to gel.

2. In a larger bowl, whisk the almond flour, arrowroot starch, sea salt, baking soda, and cinnamon. Make a well in the center of the dry ingredients, and pour in the chia seed mixture, applesauce, almond milk, and vanilla. Whisk all ingredients into a thick batter.

3. Heat butter or coconut oil on an electric griddle or heavy skillet over medium-high until sizzling. Drop 1½ tablespoons of batter per pancake onto the grill or skillet, and cook for 3–4 minutes on one side until the bottom has browned. Then flip and cook for an additional 1–2 minutes until the underside has browned. Serve hot with butter and pure maple syrup or honey.

PER SERVING: Calories: 292 | Fat: 22 g | Protein: 11 g | Sodium: 468 mg | Fiber: 6 g | Carbohydrates: 16 g | Sugar: 4 g | GI: Very low

Slow Cooker Breakfast Quinoa with Fruit

Take a break from oatmeal and try this fruity quinoa instead!

INGREDIENTS | SERVES 4

1 cup quinoa

2 cups water

½ cup dried mixed berries

1 pear, thinly sliced and peeled if desired

½ cup organic sucanat sugar

½ teaspoon ground ginger

¼ teaspoon ground cinnamon

⅛ teaspoon ground cloves

⅛ teaspoon ground nutmeg

Place all the ingredients into a 4-quart slow cooker. Stir. Cook for 2½ hours on high, or around 4 hours on low, or until the quinoa has absorbed most of the liquid and is light and fluffy.

PER SERVING: Calories: 297 | Fat: 3 g | Protein: 6.5 g | Sodium: 14 mg | Fiber: 5 g | Carbohydrates: 64 g | Sugar: 32.5 g | GI: Low

Antioxidant Fruit and Nut Salad

Fruit salad can be eaten any time, but it is particularly good for breakfast. Berries are full of antioxidants, and walnuts have one of the best omega profiles among nuts to reduce inflammation. This is a winning combination.

INGREDIENTS | SERVES 2

½ cup sliced strawberries

½ cup raspberries

½ cup blackberries

½ cup blueberries

½ cup dried mulberries

½ cup chopped walnuts

1 cup plain yogurt

Combine the berries and walnuts. Divide the yogurt into two bowls, and top with the berry and walnut mixture to serve.

PER SERVING: Calories: 357 | Fat: 24 g | Protein: 11 g | Sodium: 5.5 mg | Fiber: 8.5 g | Carbohydrates: 29.5 g | Sugar: 20 g | GI: Moderate

Easy Pancake Recipe

This pancake recipe is quick and easy and can be multiplied to make enough for an entire family. Once cooked, sprinkle the pancake with cinnamon or a small amount of agave nectar for an old-fashioned pancake taste.

INGREDIENTS | SERVES 1

1 banana
1 large egg
1 teaspoon nut butter of choice
2 teaspoons coconut oil

Bananas as Thickeners

Bananas can be a good replacement for flour. Bananas act as thickening agents in recipes that would normally be too fluid.

1. In a small bowl, mash the banana with a fork.

2. Beat the egg and add it to the banana.

3. Add the nut butter and mix well.

4. Lightly coat a large frying pan or griddle with coconut oil and pour the entire pancake mixture onto pre-heated pan.

5. Cook until lightly brown on each side, about 2 minutes per side.

PER SERVING: Calories: 389 | Fat: 17 g | Protein: 9.5 g | Sodium: 66 mg | Fiber: 7 g | Carbohydrates: 54 g | Sugar: 5 g | GI: Low

Blueberry Almond Scones

These slightly sweet scones have a light texture with a soft crumb. Try different types of fruit, such as strawberries—or even chocolate chips—in place of the blueberries.

INGREDIENTS | SERVES 8

Olive oil, as needed

3 cups blanched almond flour

¾ cup arrowroot starch or tapioca starch

½ teaspoon baking soda

¼ teaspoon sea salt

¼ cup coconut palm sugar or sugar

⅓ cup butter or coconut oil

1 large egg, slightly whisked

⅔ cup almond milk

1 teaspoon vanilla extract

½ teaspoon lemon juice or apple cider vinegar

1 cup fresh or frozen blueberries (do not defrost if frozen)

Traditional Scones versus Almond Flour Scones

Traditional scones are created by shaping the dough into a round loaf and slicing it before baking. These scones, however, are made in a cake pan and then sliced into triangles after they are cooked because almond flour dough is not quite thick enough to support itself baking without a pan. You could use a scone baking pan, but it's just as easy to bake the dough in a cake pan and then slice it.

1. Preheat the oven to 350°F. Line a 9" cake pan with parchment paper and brush with olive oil. Set aside.

2. In a large bowl, whisk the almond flour, arrowroot starch, baking soda, salt, and coconut palm sugar. Using a fork and knife or a pastry cutter, cut the butter or coconut oil evenly into the flour mixture until it resembles small peas. Set aside. In a small bowl, mix the egg, almond milk, vanilla extract, and lemon juice.

3. Mix the wet ingredients with the dry ingredients until thoroughly incorporated. Add the blueberries and mix. The batter will be thick. Pour the batter into the cake pan and smooth the top with a spatula.

4. Bake for 25–30 minutes until edges of the scone are golden brown and a toothpick inserted in the middle comes out mostly clean with few crumbs.

5. Remove the scone from the oven and set aside to cool for several minutes. Cut the round scone into 8 triangular scones.

PER SERVING: Calories: 415 | Fat: 29 g | Protein: 10 g | Sodium: 172 mg | Fiber: 5 g | Carbohydrates: 32 g | Sugar: 11 g | GI: Low

Salmon and Broccoli Stir-Fry

This is a quick and easy breakfast, in addition to being good for you.
You can blanch the broccoli in advance.

INGREDIENTS | SERVES 2

½ pound broccoli florets
½ pound salmon fillet, skin removed
1 tablespoon olive oil
1 teaspoon sesame oil
1 teaspoon minced fresh ginger
2 slices pickled ginger, chopped
1 clove garlic, minced
1 teaspoon gluten-free hoisin sauce
1 cup brown rice (optional)
5 scallions, chopped

1. Blanch the broccoli in boiling water for 5 minutes; drain.

2. Toss the broccoli and salmon over medium-high heat in a large frying pan with the olive oil and sesame oil. Cook, stirring for 3–4 minutes.

3. Add the ginger, pickled ginger, garlic, and hoisin sauce, and serve over rice, garnished with scallions.

PER SERVING: Calories: 631 | Fat: 19 g | Protein: 32 g | Sodium: 95 mg | Fiber: 7 g | Carbohydrates: 82 g | Sugar: 3 g | GI: Moderate

Food Safety

When preparing a dish that lists fish, seafood, or poultry as one of the ingredients, be sure to keep the fish, seafood, or poultry ice-cold during preparation to ensure food safety. If you will be doing a lot of handling of the ingredient or if the item will be standing on the counter for a long time, keep a bowl of ice nearby to place the ingredient in while you are tending to other steps of the recipe.

CHAPTER 15

Lunch

Turkey Lettuce Wraps

Turkey is a good protein source that kids are sure to love. Although these wraps are a bit complex to put together, you can make a larger batch of the filling and serve it over salad at a later meal.

INGREDIENTS | SERVES 4

3 tablespoons walnut oil
3 shallots, chopped
1 piece lemongrass, thinly sliced
1 serrano pepper, thinly sliced
½ teaspoon freshly ground black pepper
1½ pounds ground turkey
⅓ cup fresh lime juice
2 tablespoons sesame oil
4 tablespoons coconut oil
½ cup thinly sliced Thai basil leaves
8 large butter lettuce leaves

1. In a large skillet, heat the walnut oil over medium heat.

2. Add the shallots, lemongrass, serrano pepper, and black pepper. Cook until the shallots soften, about 4 minutes.

3. Add the ground turkey and stir frequently until cooked through, approximately 8–10 minutes.

4. Add the lime juice, sesame oil, and coconut oil and cook for 1 minute.

5. Turn the heat off and mix in the basil leaves.

6. Wrap the mixture in the lettuce leaves and serve.

PER SERVING, 2 STUFFED LETTUCE LEAVES: Calories: 381 | Fat: 29 g | Protein: 40 g | Sodium: 1 mg | Fiber: 1 g | Carbohydrates: 1 g | Sugar: 0 g | GI: Very low

Slow Cooker Mango Pork Morsels

In this recipe, the mango provides natural sweetness and a tropical flair.
Plate and pierce each piece with a toothpick.

INGREDIENTS | SERVES 10

1½ pounds pork loin, cubed

2 mangoes, cubed (see sidebar)

3 cloves garlic, minced

1 jalapeño, seeded and minced

1 tablespoon salsa

¼ teaspoon salt

¼ teaspoon freshly ground black pepper

2 teaspoons ground chipotle

1 teaspoon New Mexico chili powder

½ teaspoon oregano

2 tablespoons orange juice

2 tablespoons lime juice

1. Quickly brown the pork in a skillet over medium heat. Add the browned pork and cubed mango to a 4-quart slow cooker.

2. In a small bowl, whisk together the garlic, jalapeño, salsa, salt, pepper, chipotle, chili powder, oregano, and the orange and lime juices. Pour over the mango and pork. Stir.

3. Cook on low for 6 hours; remove the cover and cook on high for 30 minutes. Stir before serving.

PER SERVING: Calories: 32 | Fat: 0 g | Protein: 0.5 g | Sodium: 73 mg | Fiber: 1 g | Carbohydrates: 8 g | Sugar: 6.5 g | GI: Very low

How to Cut Up a Mango

Slice the mango in half vertically on either side of the large flat pit. Then, using the tip of a knife, cut vertical lines into the flesh without piercing the skin. Make horizontal lines in the flesh to form cubes. Use a spoon to scoop out the cubes. Repeat for the other side.

Mediterranean Chickpea Bake

This flavorful dish can be enjoyed as a side dish or as a main course.
Remember, always soak your fresh beans!

INGREDIENTS | SERVES 4

5 tablespoons olive oil

1 large onion, finely chopped

4 cloves garlic, minced

1 large tomato, chopped

2 teaspoons ground cumin

1 teaspoon paprika

2 large bunches fresh organic spinach, washed

2 cups cooked chickpeas

Salt and pepper to taste

1. Heat the olive oil in a medium frying pan on medium.

2. Fry the onion and garlic for 2–3 minutes, until the onion starts to become translucent; then add the tomato, cumin, and paprika. Continue cooking for 5 minutes.

3. Add the spinach and chickpeas to the pan.

4. Reduce the heat and cover with a lid. Cook, stirring frequently, until the spinach is wilted and the chickpeas are tender. Add salt and pepper to taste.

PER SERVING: Calories: 352 | Fat: 20 g | Protein: 13 g | Sodium: 587 mg | Fiber: 9 g | Carbohydrates: 35 g | Sugar: 5 g | GI: Low

Baked Chicken Wings

Cayenne pepper is known for its metabolism-boosting properties. Blended with paprika and garlic,
cayenne is sure to kick up the heat in these chicken wings.

INGREDIENTS | SERVES 4

12 chicken wings

3 tablespoons gluten-free soy sauce

½ tablespoon garlic powder

1 teaspoon paprika

1 teaspoon cayenne pepper

2 teaspoons honey

Salt and pepper to taste

1 tablespoon olive oil

1. Wash the chicken wings and pat dry.

2. Combine the remaining ingredients, except the olive oil, in a bowl. Add the wings and coat with the mixture. Cover and refrigerate for 1–2 hours or overnight.

3. Preheat the oven to 425°F. Drizzle the pan with olive oil. Place wings in one layer in the baking dish.

4. Bake for 40 minutes or until golden brown. Turn the wings over after 20 minutes to allow even cooking.

PER SERVING: Calories: 221 | Fat: 14 g | Protein: 18 g | Sodium: 2199 mg | Fiber: 0 g | Carbohydrates: 6 g | Sugar: 6 g | GI: Low

Chicken Enchiladas

If you have been craving a Mexican feast, try this spicy Paleolithic alternative.
This recipe has most of the taste of traditional enchiladas without the carbohydrates.

INGREDIENTS | SERVES 8

2 tablespoons olive oil

2 pounds boneless, skinless chicken breast, cut into 1" cubes

4 cloves garlic, minced

½ cup finely chopped onion

2 cups chopped tomatoes

1 teaspoon ground cumin

1 teaspoon chili powder

½ cup chopped fresh cilantro

Juice from 2 limes

1 (10-ounce) package frozen organic chopped spinach, thawed and drained

8 collard green leaves

1. Heat the olive oil in a medium skillet over medium-high heat. Sauté chicken, garlic, and onion in the hot oil until thoroughly cooked, about 10 minutes.

2. Add tomatoes, cumin, chili powder, cilantro, and lime juice, and simmer for 5 minutes.

3. Add the spinach and simmer for 5 more minutes. Remove from heat.

4. In a separate large pot, quickly steam the collard greens with a little water to soften them, about 3 minutes.

5. Wrap the chicken mixture in the collard greens and serve.

PER SERVING: Calories: 151 | Fat: 5.5 g | Protein: 22 g | Sodium: 35 mg | Fiber: 2 g | Carbohydrates: 5 g | Sugar: 3 g | GI: Low

Shredded Chicken Wraps

Wraps are a great way to get the feel of a tortilla wrap without the forbidden carbohydrates. You can easily substitute your favorite meat or fish for the chicken to vary your lunchtime menu.

INGREDIENTS | SERVES 8

2 boneless, skinless chicken breasts, cooked (baked or pan fried)
2 celery stalks, chopped
¼ cup chopped basil
2 tablespoons olive oil
2 tablespoons lemon juice
1 teaspoon minced garlic
Freshly ground black pepper to taste
1 head radicchio or romaine lettuce

1. Shred or finely chop the chicken and place it in a medium bowl.

2. Mix chicken with celery, basil, olive oil, lemon juice, garlic, and pepper.

3. Separate the lettuce leaves and place on eight plates.

4. Spoon the chicken mixture onto the lettuce leaves and roll them up.

PER SERVING: Calories: 133 | Fat: 4 g | Protein: 9 g | Sodium: 14 mg | Fiber: 0.5 g | Carbohydrates: 1 g | Sugar: 0 g | GI: Very low

Curried Shrimp with Veggies

This curried shrimp and vegetable dish is quick and easy, but quite authentic-tasting. It is sure to please everyone in your family who is fond of Indian cuisine.

INGREDIENTS | SERVES 4

2 tablespoons olive oil
1 tablespoon green curry powder
1 pound medium or large shrimp, peeled and deveined
1 (12-ounce) bag organic frozen broccoli florets
4 large carrots, peeled and sliced
1 (8-ounce) can coconut milk

1. In a large skillet over medium heat, warm the olive oil and green curry powder.

2. Add the shrimp, broccoli, carrots, and coconut milk.

3. Cook until all vegetables are tender and the coconut milk cooks down to a thick, paste-like consistency (approximately 15 minutes).

PER SERVING: Calories: 343 | Fat: 21 g | Protein: 22 g | Sodium: 250 mg | Fiber: 6 g | Carbohydrates: 21 g | Sugar: 4.5 g | GI: Moderate

Haddock Fish Cakes

These familiar fish cakes have the fresh flavor of haddock.
Serve them with a spicy sauce or a fresh spritz of lemon.

INGREDIENTS | SERVES 6

1 pound haddock

2 medium leeks, trimmed and diced

1 medium organic red bell pepper, seeded and diced

2 eggs

Freshly cracked black pepper to taste

1 tablespoon olive oil

1. Finely shred the raw fish with a fork. Combine all the ingredients except the oil in a medium bowl; mix well. Form the mixture into small oval patties.

2. Heat the oil in a medium sauté pan over medium-high heat. Place the haddock in the pan and loosely cover with the lid; sauté the fish cakes for 4–6 minutes on each side. Drain on a rack covered with paper towels; serve immediately.

PER SERVING: Calories: 107 | Fat: 4 g | Protein: 13.5 g | Sodium: 67 mg | Fiber: 1 g | Carbohydrates: 5 g | Sugar: 0 g | GI: Very low

Salmon Skewers

Salmon has a wonderful omega profile,
being one of the highest sources of omega-3 fatty acids.

INGREDIENTS | SERVES 4

8 ounces salmon fillet

1 medium red onion, peeled and cut into wedges

2 medium red bell peppers, seeded and cut into 2" squares

12 mushrooms

12 cherry tomatoes

1. Preheat grill to 350°F. Cut the salmon into 1"–2" cubes.

2. Thread all the ingredients on metal skewers, alternating the vegetables and meat.

3. Grill over medium-high heat until vegetables are soft and the salmon is light pink, about 10 minutes, depending on the thickness of the salmon steak.

PER SERVING: Calories: 107 | Fat: 3.5 g | Protein: 15 g | Sodium: 235 mg | Fiber: 2.5 g | Carbohydrates: 6.5 g | Sugar: 6 g | GI: Low

Mackerel with Tomato and Cucumber Salad

According to the USDA National Nutrient Database, mackerel contains 2.3 grams of omega-3 for every 100 grams of fish. That makes mackerel the highest EFA (essential fatty acid)-containing fish.

INGREDIENTS | SERVES 4

15 ounces mackerel fillets, drained
1 clove garlic, crushed
1½ tablespoons olive oil
1 tablespoon chopped fresh basil
½ teaspoon freshly ground black pepper
10 cherry tomatoes, halved
½ cucumber, peeled and diced
1 small onion, peeled and chopped
2 cups mixed lettuce greens

1. Place the mackerel in a medium bowl with the garlic and olive oil.

2. Add the basil and pepper to the mackerel mixture and place in a medium frying pan. Sauté over medium heat for 5–8 minutes each side, or until brown.

3. Cut the cooked mackerel into bite-size pieces and add to a large serving bowl.

4. Stir in the cherry tomatoes, cucumber, onion, and lettuce, and serve.

PER SERVING: Calories: 240 | Fat: 17 g | Protein: 16 g | Sodium: 82 mg | Fiber: 1 g | Carbohydrates: 3.5 g | Sugar: 1 g | GI: Low

Mahi-Mahi Tacos with Avocado

These California-style tacos can be prepared with any meaty, mild fish or shrimp.

INGREDIENTS | SERVES 4

1 pound mahi-mahi
Salt and pepper to taste
1 teaspoon olive oil
1 avocado
4 sprouted corn tortillas
2 cups shredded cabbage
2 limes, quartered

1. Season the fish with salt and pepper. Heat the oil in a large frying pan on medium. Once the oil is hot, sauté the fish for about 3–4 minutes on each side. Slice or flake the fish into 1-ounce pieces.

2. Slice the avocado in half. Remove the seed and, using a spoon, remove the flesh intact from the skin. Slice the avocado halves into ½"-thick slices.

3. In a small pan, warm the corn tortillas; cook for about 1 minute on each side.

4. Place ¼ of the mahi-mahi on each tortilla; top with the avocado and cabbage. Serve with lime wedges.

PER SERVING: Calories: 251 | Fat: 9 g | Protein: 25 g | Sodium: 889 mg | Fiber: 6 g | Carbohydrates: 21 g | Sugar: 2.5 g | GI: Low

Jambalaya

This authentic Louisiana favorite is full of flavor and spice.

INGREDIENTS | SERVES 6

1 tablespoon olive oil

2 boneless, skinless (optional) chicken breasts, chopped

8 ounces andouille sausage, sliced

12 medium shrimp, peeled and deveined

½ medium onion, peeled and chopped

2 medium organic green bell peppers, seeded and chopped

2 stalks celery, diced

2 cloves garlic, minced

¼ teaspoon crushed red pepper

1 teaspoon chili powder

2 teaspoons dried oregano

Freshly ground black pepper to taste

6 ounces brown rice

1 (32-ounce) box gluten-free chicken broth or homemade stock

1 can diced tomatoes

1 cup water

Tabasco to taste

1. Pour the oil into a large pot and place on medium-high heat. Sauté the chicken and sausage until browned, about 6–8 minutes. Add the shrimp; cook and stir until shrimp are opaque, about 4 minutes.

2. Add the onion, bell pepper, celery, and garlic; season with crushed red pepper, chili powder, oregano, and black pepper. Cook until the onion is tender.

3. Stir in the rice, broth, tomatoes, and water. Bring to a boil and then reduce heat; simmer until the rice is cooked. Stir in the Tabasco before serving.

PER SERVING: Calories: 328 | Fat: 14 g | Protein: 22 g | Sodium: 906 mg | Fiber: 3 g | Carbohydrates: 29 g | Sugar: 3 g | GI: Moderate

Slow Cooker Dijon Beef Roast

Dijon mustard gives this roast a delicious tangy flavor. This recipe is perfect for roast beef sandwiches or for a traditional Sunday meal with mashed potatoes and gravy.

INGREDIENTS | SERVES 6

1 large onion, peeled and thickly sliced
1 (3–4 pound) beef round roast
3–4 tablespoons Dijon mustard
½ teaspoon salt
½ teaspoon freshly ground black pepper
1 tablespoon olive oil
½ cup gluten-free or homemade beef broth, or water

1. Place the onion slices in a greased 4-quart slow cooker.

2. Rub the beef roast with the Dijon mustard. Place it on top of the sliced onions.

3. Sprinkle salt and pepper on top of beef roast and drizzle with the olive oil and beef broth.

4. Cover and cook on high for 2½–3 hours or on low for 5–6 hours. Cooking time will vary depending on your preference of doneness (either rare, medium, or well done). For a rarer roast, check the internal temperature (around 145°F) after cooking for 1½ hours on high or 3 hours on low. Serve the roast with the cooked onions and au jus drizzled on top.

PER SERVING: Calories: 499 | Fat: 24 g | Protein: 54 g | Sodium: 346 mg | Fiber: 1 g | Carbohydrates: 3 g | Sugar: 1 g | GI: Very low

Slow Cooker Hatteras Clam Chowder

This cozy, creamy chowder is thickened only by potatoes. Serve it with a fresh green salad and homemade gluten-free bread.

INGREDIENTS | SERVES 4

4 slices bacon, diced
1 small onion, peeled and diced
2 medium russet potatoes, peeled and diced
1 (8-ounce) bottle clam stock
2–3 cups water
½ teaspoon salt
½ teaspoon freshly ground black pepper
2 (6.5-ounce) cans minced clams, with juice

1. In a 2-quart or larger saucepan, sauté the bacon over medium-high heat until crispy and browned. Add the onion and sauté until translucent, about 3–5 minutes. Add the cooked onions and bacon to a greased 2.5-quart slow cooker.

2. Add the potatoes, clam stock, and enough water to cover (2–3 cups). Add salt and pepper.

3. Cover and cook on high for 3 hours until the potatoes are very tender.

4. One hour before serving, add clams along with broth and cook until heated through.

PER SERVING: Calories: 253 | Fat: 11.5 g | Protein: 12.5 g | Sodium: 601 mg | Fiber: 2 g | Carbohydrates: 25 g | Sugar: 3 g | GI: Low

CHAPTER 16

Dinner

Paleo Spaghetti

This is a great alternative to traditional pasta. Serve with sauce and turkey meatballs for a great Paleolithic take on Nonno's spaghetti and meatball recipe!

INGREDIENTS | SERVES 4

1 large spaghetti squash

Pasta Alternative

Spaghetti squash is a fantastic carbohydrate source for all you pasta addicts out there. This squash looks like spaghetti when the meat is peeled from the skin. It has the relative texture of pasta. And, most important, it is quite filling.

1. Preheat the oven to 350°F.

2. Cut the squash in half lengthwise.

3. Place cut-side down in a baking dish with ¼" water.

4. Cook 30 minutes, turn the squash over, and cook until it is soft all the way through, approximately 10 minutes.

5. Shred with a fork. Serve with your favorite sauce.

PER SERVING: Calories: 94 | Fat: 0 g | Protein: 2 g | Sodium: 1.5 mg | Fiber: 0 g | Carbohydrates: 20 g | Sugar: 4 g | GI: Low

Poached Mediterranean Chicken

Poaching a skinless, boneless chicken breast is a calorie-conscious and practical mode of cooking. The chicken does not dry out as it does when grilled or broiled, and no oil is necessary.

INGREDIENTS | SERVES 2

1 cup low-salt chicken broth or homemade stock

1 large fresh tomato, cored and chopped

4 ounces pearl onions, fresh or frozen

4–6 cloves Roasted Garlic (see recipe sidebar)

10 spicy black olives, such as kalamata or Sicilian

10 green olives, pitted (no pimientos)

½ teaspoon dried, crumbled oregano leaves

1 teaspoon dried, crumbled mint leaves

4 fresh basil leaves, torn

2 (4-ounce) boneless, skinless chicken breasts

Salt and pepper to taste

½ teaspoon lemon zest

4 sprigs parsley

1. Make the poaching liquid by placing all of the ingredients except for the chicken, salt and pepper, lemon zest, and parsley in a large saucepan. Bring to a boil; reduce heat and simmer for 5 minutes.

2. Add the chicken, salt, and pepper. Simmer for another 8 minutes and add the lemon zest. Sprinkle with parsley and serve.

PER SERVING: Calories: 370 | Fat: 14 g | Protein: 43 g | Sodium: 1523 mg | Fiber: 3 g | Carbohydrates: 11 g | Sugar: 4 g | GI: Zero

How to Make Roasted Garlic

You can easily make your own roasted garlic in the oven. Simply place 2–4 whole (unpeeled) heads of garlic in a pan. Drizzle 2 tablespoons of olive oil over the garlic and bake at 350°F for about 45 minutes. Allow to cool for 5–10 minutes and then gently squeeze garlic cloves out of the "paper" surrounding them. Use in any recipe calling for roasted garlic or even spread on your favorite vegetables!

Lemon Chicken

A classic citrus chicken with fresh herbs. It has the perfect amount of lemon, so it's not too sour.

INGREDIENTS | SERVES 6

⅓ cup lemon juice

2 tablespoons lemon zest

3 cloves garlic, minced

2 tablespoons chopped fresh thyme

2 tablespoons chopped fresh rosemary

2 tablespoons olive oil

1 teaspoon salt

1 teaspoon freshly ground black pepper

3 pounds bone-in chicken thighs

1. To make the marinade, combine the lemon juice, lemon zest, garlic, thyme, rosemary, olive oil, salt, and pepper in a small bowl. Place the chicken in a large bowl and pour the marinade on top. Let marinate in the refrigerator for 2 hours.

2. Preheat the oven to 425°F. Place the marinated chicken in one layer in a large baking dish. Spoon the leftover marinade over the chicken.

3. Bake until the chicken is completely cooked through, about 50 minutes. The internal temperature will be 175°F.

PER SERVING: Calories: 254 | Fat: 19 g | Protein: 16 g | Sodium: 308 mg | Fiber: 0 g | Carbohydrates: 4 g | Sugar: 0 g | GI: Very low

Roast Turkey

Enjoy this signature main course for a holiday meal or a special family dinner.

INGREDIENTS | SERVES 8

1 (8-pound) turkey
10 cloves garlic, crushed
1 bunch fresh tarragon, chopped
⅓ cup olive oil
Salt and pepper to taste

1. Heat the oven to 450°F. Place the turkey breast-side down on a large cutting board and remove the backbone. Turn it over and place it breast-side up in a large roasting pan.

2. Arrange the garlic and tarragon under the turkey and in the crevices of the wings and legs. Drizzle the turkey with olive oil and season with salt and pepper.

3. Roast for 20 minutes, remove from the oven, turn the oven down to 400°F, baste the turkey with the juices, and return to the oven.

4. Cook until the internal temperature of the turkey is 165°F–170°F on a meat thermometer, generally about 3–3½ hours for an 8-pound turkey. Let the turkey rest before carving.

PER SERVING: Calories: 190 | Fat: 10 g | Protein: 24 g | Sodium: 311 mg | Fiber: 0 g | Carbohydrates: 1 g | Sugar: 0 g | GI: Very low

Grilled Jerk Chicken

This marinated chicken dish is great to make in large quantities for eating throughout the week. It is a fantastic summer dish to cook outside on the grill.

INGREDIENTS | SERVES 4

5 cloves chopped garlic

1 teaspoon ground ginger

1 teaspoon dried thyme

1 teaspoon ground paprika

1 teaspoon ground cinnamon

½ teaspoon ground allspice

½ cup lemon juice

½ cup red wine

4 boneless chicken breasts

1. Preheat oven to 375°F.

2. Combine the garlic, ginger, thyme, paprika, cinnamon, allspice, lemon juice, and red wine in a large bowl.

3. Add the chicken and marinate for at least 5 hours in the refrigerator.

4. Prepare a charcoal or gas grill.

5. Remove the chicken from marinade and place on a baking pan, in the oven. Discard marinade. Cook for 25 minutes or until chicken is cooked throughout.

PER SERVING: Calories: 181 | Fat: 2.5 g | Protein: 35 g | Sodium: 0.5 mg | Fiber: 0 g | Carbohydrates: 2 g | Sugar: 2 g | GI: Low

Duck Breast with Mushroom Sauce over Wild Rice or Polenta

If you know a mycologist or visit some farmers' markets, you can get wonderful wild mushrooms. Otherwise, use the shiitakes or brown mushrooms available in the supermarket.

INGREDIENTS | SERVES 2

2 boneless duck breasts

2 tablespoons brown rice flour or almond flour

Salt and pepper to taste

½ teaspoon dried thyme

⅛ teaspoon ground cayenne

½ teaspoon Chinese five-spice powder

2 tablespoons olive oil

1 tablespoon butter

4 shallots

1 cup coarsely chopped wild or exotic mushrooms

½ cup gluten-free chicken broth or homemade stock

2 tablespoons Calvados (French apple brandy)

1 tablespoon fresh rosemary, or 1 teaspoon dried

1 cup wild rice, prepared to package directions

1. Coat the duck breasts in a mixture of flour, salt, pepper, thyme, cayenne, and five-spice powder. In a large frying pan, heat the olive oil over medium heat and sauté the duck for 4–5 minutes per side to brown.

2. Remove the duck to a warm serving platter.

3. Using the same pan, stir in the butter and shallots. Sauté for 3–4 minutes. Add the mushrooms and toss to coat with butter.

4. Stir in the chicken broth, Calvados, and rosemary. Return the duck to the pan. Cover and cook for 5 minutes.

5. Serve the duck with mushroom sauce over the wild rice.

PER SERVING: Calories: 680 | Fat: 31 g | Protein: 36 g | Sodium: 1279 mg | Fiber: 4 g | Carbohydrates: 51 g | Sugar: 3 g | GI: Moderate

Lamb Meatballs

Meatballs are always a kid favorite. These grass-fed lamb meatballs are high in good fats that contribute to their taste and their health factor.

INGREDIENTS | SERVES 6

¼ cup pine nuts
4 tablespoons olive oil, divided
1½ pounds ground grass-fed lamb
¼ cup minced garlic
2 tablespoons ground cumin

1. Over medium-high heat in a medium frying pan, sauté the pine nuts in 2 tablespoons of olive oil for 2 minutes until brown. Remove them from the pan and allow them to cool.

2. In a large bowl, combine the lamb, garlic, cumin, and pine nuts, and form the mixture into meatballs.

3. Add the remaining olive oil to the pan and fry the meatballs until cooked through, about 5–10 minutes, depending on size of meatballs.

PER SERVING: Calories: 148 | Fat: 13 g | Protein: 5 g | Sodium: 201 mg | Fiber: 2.5 g | Carbohydrates: 6.5 g | Sugar: 1 g | GI: Very low

Beef Tenderloin with Chimichurri

This is simple enough to make for a weeknight meal or perfect for a sophisticated gourmet dinner party.

INGREDIENTS | SERVES 2

1 cup parsley
3 cloves garlic
¼ cup capers, drained
2 tablespoons red wine vinegar
1 teaspoon Dijon mustard
2 tablespoons olive oil
Salt and pepper to taste
2 (5-ounce) beef tenderloins

1. In a small bowl whisk together parsley, garlic, capers, vinegar, mustard, and oil. Season with salt and pepper as desired.

2. Heat grill to 350°F. Grill the steaks to medium-rare, about 4–5 minutes per side. Serve hot.

PER SERVING: Calories: 435 | Fat: 30 g | Protein: 37 g | Sodium: 1299 mg | Fiber: 1 g | Carbohydrates: 4 g | Sugar: 1 g | GI: Very low

Beef Brisket with Onions and Mushrooms

This roast is packed with flavor and so tender that it will melt in your mouth.

INGREDIENTS | SERVES 4

2 cloves garlic

½ teaspoon salt, plus more to taste

4 tablespoons olive oil, divided

½ bunch rosemary, chopped

1 pound beef brisket

Freshly ground black pepper to taste

3 large onions, peeled and quartered

3 cups sliced white mushrooms

3 celery stalks, cut into large chunks

2 cups dry red cooking wine

1 (16-ounce) can whole tomatoes, chopped

2 bay leaves

Kitchen Gadgets

The mortar and pestle was originally used in pharmacies to crush ingredients to make medicines. In the culinary world, the mortar and pestle is a very useful tool for crushing seeds and nuts and making guacamole, pesto, and garlic paste.

1. Preheat the oven to 325°F.

2. Place the garlic, ½ teaspoon salt, 2 tablespoons oil, and chopped rosemary leaves in a mortar or a bowl and, using a pestle or the back of a spoon, mash them to make a paste.

3. Season the brisket with salt and pepper. Heat the remaining olive oil in a large frying pan, place the brisket in the pan, and sear it over medium-high to make a dark crust on both sides. Place the brisket in a large roasting pan and spread the rosemary paste on it. Place the onions, mushrooms, and celery around the brisket in the pan. Pour the wine and tomatoes over the top and toss in the bay leaves.

4. Tightly cover the pan with foil and place it in the oven. Bake for about 4 hours, basting with pan juices every 30 minutes, until the beef is very tender.

5. Let the brisket rest for 15 minutes before slicing it across the grain at a slight diagonal. Remove the bay leaves before serving.

PER SERVING: Calories: 633 | Fat: 39 g | Protein: 25 g | Sodium: 1548 mg | Fiber: 3 g | Carbohydrates: 26 g | Sugar: 15 g | GI: Low

Pork Chops with Balsamic Glaze

Shallots, balsamic vinegar, and agave nectar add a balanced touch of sweetness to this savory dish.

INGREDIENTS | SERVES 4

4 (5-ounce) center-cut pork chops
1 teaspoon salt, divided
Freshly ground black pepper to taste
2 tablespoons olive oil
6 large shallots, peeled and quartered
½ cup balsamic vinegar
2 teaspoons honey

1. Wash and pat dry the pork chops. Season them with ½ teaspoon salt and pepper.

2. Heat the oil in a large frying pan on medium-high heat. Add the pork and shallots to the pan. Turn the pork over once, to cook about 3 minutes on each side, and stir the shallots occasionally until tender, about 3 minutes. Transfer the pork to a plate, cover it, and set it aside.

3. Add the vinegar, honey, ½ teaspoon salt, and a pinch of pepper to the shallots in the pan. Cook until the liquid begins to thicken, about 1–2 minutes.

4. Turn the heat down to medium-low, return the pork to the pan, and coat the pork well with the sauce. Cook for 3–4 minutes; a thermometer inserted into the pork should read 150°F.

5. Remove the pork from the pan, turn the heat up, and allow the remaining sauce to thicken. Pour the sauce over the pork chops before serving.

PER SERVING: Calories: 288 | Fat: 12 g | Protein: 30 g | Sodium: 642 mg | Fiber: 0 g | Carbohydrates: 10 g | Sugar: 6 g | GI: Very low

Grilled Rib Lamb Chops with Garlic and Citrus

Young lamb is a great party dish and is perfect when cooked medium-rare.

INGREDIENTS | SERVES 2

2 teaspoons olive oil

Juice and zest from ½ lemon

1 tablespoon grapefruit juice

1–2 cloves garlic, minced

1 teaspoon dried rosemary, or 1 tablespoon fresh

Salt and pepper to taste

8 baby rib lamb chops, about ½" each, well trimmed

2 tablespoons white vermouth, for basting

1. Using a mortar and pestle, mash together the olive oil, lemon juice and zest, grapefruit juice, garlic, rosemary, salt, and pepper.

2. Coat the lamb chops with the garlic mixture and let rest in the refrigerator for 1 hour.

3. Heat the grill to high. Place the chops over a high flame until they are seared on one side. Baste with the vermouth and turn after 3 minutes. Baste again and reduce the heat. Cover the grill and let the chops roast for 8 minutes.

PER SERVING: Calories: 513 | Fat: 24 g | Protein: 68 g | Sodium: 1199 mg | Fiber: 0 g | Carbohydrates: 0 g | Sugar: 0 g | GI: Zero

Easy Slow Cooker Leg of Lamb

Although lamb can be an expensive cut of meat, it is often on sale during the holidays. Stock up on several cuts and freeze them when you find good prices.

INGREDIENTS | SERVES 6

1 (4-pound) bone-in leg of lamb

5 cloves garlic, skin removed, cut into spears

2 tablespoons olive oil

1 tablespoon dried rosemary

½ teaspoon salt

½ teaspoon freshly ground black pepper

4 cups low-sodium, gluten-free chicken stock

¼ cup gluten-free soy sauce or red wine

1. Make small incisions evenly in the lamb. Place the garlic spears into the small openings.

2. Rub the olive oil, rosemary, salt, and pepper over the lamb. Place the lamb into a greased 4- or 6-quart slow cooker.

3. Pour the stock and soy sauce (or wine) around the lamb. Cook on high for 4 hours or on low for 8 hours.

4. Serve the roast lamb in bowls. Ladle the sauce from the slow cooker over each serving.

PER SERVING: Calories: 536 | Fat: 24 g | Protein: 66 g | Sodium: 1195 mg | Fiber: 1 g | Carbohydrates: 8 g | Sugar: 3 g | GI: Very low

Grilled Trout

Cooking the fish inside the foil packets keeps it tender and moist.

INGREDIENTS | SERVES 2

2 whole trout, heads removed, cleaned and butterflied

1 teaspoon freshly ground black pepper

2 cloves garlic, minced

½ teaspoon chopped fresh rosemary

1 teaspoon chopped fresh parsley

6 sprigs fresh rosemary

1 lemon, halved; one half thinly sliced

1. Preheat the oven to 350°F. Place the trout in a baking dish.

2. Season both sides of trout with pepper, garlic, chopped rosemary, and parsley.

3. Fold the fish closed and top with the rosemary sprigs and a few slices of lemon.

4. Squeeze the lemon half over each fish.

5. Bake the fish for 15–18 until the fish is flaky.

PER SERVING: Calories: 176 | Fat: 8 g | Protein: 25 g | Sodium: 62 mg | Fiber: 0 g | Carbohydrates: 0 g | Sugar: 1 g | GI: Zero

Lemon-Garlic Shrimp and Vegetables

The shrimp will sing in this light stir-fry with hints of sweet and sour flavors.

INGREDIENTS | SERVES 2

2 tablespoons gluten-free soy sauce

1 teaspoon lemon zest

1½ tablespoons lemon juice

½ teaspoon honey

½ cup water

Freshly ground black pepper to taste

1 celery stalk, sliced

1 cup shredded red cabbage

½ medium red bell pepper, seeded and thinly sliced

3 cloves garlic, chopped

½ cup bean sprouts

1 teaspoon sesame oil

½ pound raw shrimp, peeled and deveined

1. Mix the soy sauce, lemon zest, lemon juice, honey, water, and pepper in a small bowl; set aside.

2. Brush a large frying pan with olive oil. Place the pan over medium heat.

3. Add the celery and cabbage to the pan; sauté for 1 minute. Add the bell pepper, garlic, and bean sprouts, and sauté until all vegetables are crisp-tender. Transfer the vegetables to a plate and cover.

4. Add the sesame oil to the pan. Once the oil is hot, place the shrimp in the pan and cook until they are opaque. Return the vegetables to the pan with the cooked shrimp.

5. Pour the soy sauce mixture over the shrimp and vegetables and cook for 3–4 minutes, until the sauce has reduced.

PER SERVING: Calories: 197 | Fat: 4.5 g | Protein: 26 g | Sodium: 1094 mg | Fiber: 2 g | Carbohydrates: 12 g | Sugar: 4.5 g | GI: Very low

Rotisserie-Style Chicken

Here is a delicious alternative to buying rotisserie chicken in your grocery store. This flavorful roast chicken is incredibly easy to make in your slow cooker. For a fast weeknight meal, cook the chicken overnight in the slow cooker and serve for dinner the next day.

INGREDIENTS | SERVES 6

1 (4-pound) whole chicken
1½ teaspoons salt
2 teaspoons paprika
½ teaspoon onion powder
½ teaspoon dried thyme
½ teaspoon dried basil
½ teaspoon white pepper
½ teaspoon ground cayenne pepper
½ teaspoon freshly ground black pepper
½ teaspoon garlic powder
2 tablespoons olive oil

Gravy

If you would like to make a gravy to go with the chicken, follow these directions: After removing the cooked chicken, turn the slow cooker on high. Whisk ⅓ cup of arrowroot flour or ⅓ cup of brown rice flour into the cooking juices. Add salt and pepper to taste and cook for 10–15 minutes, whisking occasionally, until the gravy has thickened. Spoon the gravy over the chicken.

1. Rinse the chicken in cold water and pat dry with a paper towel.

2. In a small bowl, mix the salt, paprika, onion powder, thyme, basil, white pepper, cayenne pepper, black pepper, and garlic powder.

3. Rub the spice mixture over the entire chicken. Rub part of the spice mixture underneath the skin, making sure to leave the skin intact.

4. Place the spice-rubbed chicken in a greased 6-quart slow cooker. Drizzle olive oil evenly over the chicken. Cook on high for 3–3½ hours or on low for 4–5 hours.

5. Remove chicken carefully from the slow cooker and place on a large plate or serving platter.

PER SERVING: Calories: 171 | Fat: 7.5 g | Protein: 23 g | Sodium: 474 mg | Fiber: 0 g | Carbohydrates: 0 g | Sugar: 0 g | GI: Very low

Mexican Pork Roast

This slow-cooked pork is an excellent main dish and can serve as a low-glycemic version of tacos. Try serving it topped with chopped tomatoes, shredded lettuce, shredded cheese, salsa, and sour cream!

INGREDIENTS | SERVES 4

1 tablespoon olive oil

1 large sweet onion, peeled and sliced

1 medium carrot, peeled and finely diced

1 jalapeño, seeded and minced

1 clove garlic, peeled and minced

½ teaspoon salt

¼ teaspoon dried Mexican oregano

¼ teaspoon ground coriander

¼ teaspoon freshly ground black pepper

1 (3-pound) pork shoulder or butt roast

1 cup gluten-free chicken broth or homemade stock

Pork and Sweet Potatoes?

Another low-glycemic meal option is to serve this pork over cooked butternut squash or mashed sweet potatoes. Serve with steamed broccoli or asparagus, along with a side of slow-cooked black beans.

1. Add the olive oil, onion, carrot, and jalapeño to a 4- to 6-quart slow cooker. Stir to coat the vegetables in the oil. Cover and cook on high for 30 minutes or until the onions are softened. Stir in the garlic.

2. In a small bowl, combine the salt, oregano, coriander, and black pepper. Rub the spice mixture onto the pork roast.

3. Add the rubbed pork roast to the slow cooker. Add the chicken broth. Cover and cook on low for 6 hours or until the pork is tender and pulls apart easily.

4. Use a slotted spoon to remove the pork and vegetables to a serving platter. Cover and let rest for 10 minutes.

5. Increase the temperature of the slow cooker to high. Cook and reduce the pan juices by half.

6. Use 2 forks to shred the pork and mix it in with the cooked onion and jalapeño. Ladle the reduced pan juices over the pork.

PER SERVING: Calories: 576 | Fat: 28 g | Protein: 67 g | Sodium: 824 mg | Fiber: 1 g | Carbohydrates: 8 g | Sugar: 2 g | GI: Very low

CHAPTER 17

Sauces, Dips, and Marinades

Red Pepper Coulis

Coulis can be made using any fruit or vegetable.
For variety, experiment by adding herbs and spices.

INGREDIENTS | SERVES 8

6 medium organic red bell peppers
1 tablespoon olive oil
Freshly cracked black pepper to taste

1. Preheat oven to 375°F.

2. Toss the red peppers with the oil in a medium bowl. Place the peppers on a racked sheet pan and put in the oven for 15–20 minutes, until the skins begin to blister and the red peppers wilt.

3. Remove them from the oven and immediately place the red peppers in a glass or ceramic container with a top. Let the peppers sit for approximately 5 minutes, and then peel off the skin. Stem, seed, and dice the peppers.

4. Place the peppers in a blender and purée until smooth. Season with black pepper.

PER SERVING: Calories: 39 | Fat: 1.5 g | Protein: 0.5 g | Sodium: 1.5 mg | Fiber: 1.5 g | Carbohydrates: 6 g | Sugar: 1 g | GI: Very low

Walnut-Parsley Pesto

Walnuts add a significant blast of omega-3 fatty acids to this delicious pesto.

INGREDIENTS | SERVES 4

½ cup walnuts
8 cloves garlic
1 bunch parsley, roughly chopped
¼ cup olive oil
Freshly cracked black pepper to taste

Pesto for All

Pesto is a generic term for anything made by pounding. Most people are familiar with traditional pesto, which is made with basil and pine nuts, but many prefer this variation with parsley and walnuts.

1. Chop the walnuts in a food processor or blender. Add the garlic and process to form a paste. Add the parsley; pulse into the walnut mixture.

2. While the blender is running, drizzle in the oil until the mixture is smooth. Add pepper to taste.

PER SERVING: Calories: 229 | Fat: 23 g | Protein: 3 g | Sodium: 6 mg | Fiber: 1 g | Carbohydrates: 4 g | Sugar: 0 g | GI: Very low

Balsamic Vinaigrette and Marinade

Because balsamic vinegar is very sweet, it needs a slightly sour counterpoint. In this recipe, it's lemon juice. It also needs a bit of zip, like pepper or mustard. Use this vinaigrette as a dressing or a marinade

INGREDIENTS | MAKES 1 CUP

2 cloves garlic, minced
2 shallots, minced
⅓ cup balsamic vinegar
Juice of ½ lemon
Salt and pepper to taste
½ teaspoon Dijon-style mustard
½ cup olive oil

Place all the ingredients except the olive oil in a blender. With the blender running on a medium setting, slowly pour the oil into the jar. Blend until very smooth. Cover and store in the refrigerator for up to 7 days.

PER SERVING (2 TABLESPOONS): Calories: 76 | Fat: 7 g | Protein: 0 g | Sodium: 150 mg | Fiber: 0 g | Carbohydrates: 2 g | Sugar: 2 g | GI: Zero

Creamy-Crunchy Avocado Dip with Red Onions and Macadamia Nuts

This is one of the best dips you can make. Try it with bagel chips, pita toast, or even good corn chips.

INGREDIENTS | SERVES 2

1 large ripe avocado, peeled, pit removed

Juice of ½ fresh lime

2 tablespoons minced red onion

2 tablespoons chopped macadamia nuts

1 teaspoon Tabasco or other hot red pepper sauce

Salt to taste

Using a small bowl, mash the avocado and mix in the rest of the ingredients. Serve chilled.

PER SERVING: Calories: 229 | Fat: 22 g | Protein: 3 g | Sodium: 150 mg | Fiber: 0 g | Carbohydrates: 10 g | Sugar: 1 g | GI: Very low

Lemon-Dill Dressing

This traditional dressing is best used on fish.

INGREDIENTS | SERVES 2

2 tablespoons olive oil

Juice of 1 lemon

1 teaspoon fresh dill

½ teaspoon freshly ground black pepper

Combine all the ingredients, mix well, and serve on salad.

PER SERVING: Calories: 120 | Fat: 14 g | Protein: 0 g | Sodium: 0.5 g | Fiber: 0 g | Carbohydrates: 0 g | Sugar: 0 g | GI: Zero

Oils

Feel free to experiment with different oils in your salad dressing. Every oil has a different flavor and fat profile. Flaxseed oil is higher in omega-3 fatty acid than others. Walnut oil has a higher omega-3 to omega-6 ratio compared with others. Udo's oil is a nice blend of oils with various omega-3s, -6s, and -9s. These oils have a nice flavor and have the best to offer in a fat profile.

Homemade Hummus

Garlic lovers can add more garlic to this popular Middle Eastern dip. You can buy hummus at the store, but this recipe is easy to make and much cheaper.

INGREDIENTS | SERVES 12

2 cups cooked chickpeas

2 cloves garlic, chopped, or more to taste

½ small white onion, peeled and chopped

1 teaspoon Tabasco or other hot sauce

½ cup fresh flat-leaf parsley or cilantro, tightly packed

Salt and pepper to taste

½ cup olive oil

Vegetable sticks, such as carrots, celery, or cucumber

Blend all the ingredients in the food processor or blender. Do not purée; the hummus should have a coarse consistency. Serve with vegetable sticks.

PER SERVING: Calories: 128 | Fat: 9 g | Protein: 2 g | Sodium: 150 mg | Fiber: 4 g | Carbohydrates: 9 g | Sugar: 2 g | GI: Low

Mint Chimichurri Sauce

Instead of the traditional mint jelly, use this mint chimichurri sauce to make a lamb recipe extra-special.

INGREDIENTS | MAKES 2 CUPS

2 cups fresh parsley

2 cups fresh cilantro

1 cup fresh mint

¾ cup olive oil

3 tablespoons red wine vinegar

Juice of 1 lemon

3 cloves garlic, minced

1 large shallot, quartered

1 teaspoon salt

1 small jalapeño, seeded and chopped

1. Wash the herbs, remove the stems, and chop the leaves.

2. In a blender, combine the olive oil, vinegar, lemon juice, garlic, shallots, salt, and jalapeño. Blend the ingredients. Add the parsley, cilantro, and mint to the blender in batches and blend until the sauce is smooth.

PER SERVING (2 TABLESPOONS): Calories: 98 | Fat: 10 g | Protein: 0 g | Sodium: 98 mg | Fiber: 1 g | Carbohydrates: 2 g | Sugar: 1 g | GI: Very low

Hollandaise Sauce

If you make Hollandaise Sauce in the blender or food processor, your sauce will not curdle.

INGREDIENTS | MAKES ¾ CUP

4 ounces sweet unsalted butter

1 whole egg

1 egg yolk

¼ teaspoon dry mustard

Juice of ½ lemon

⅛ teaspoon cayenne pepper

Salt to taste

Béarnaise Sauce and Sauce Maltaise

If you substitute white wine vinegar for lemon juice and add chives in this recipe, you will have béarnaise sauce, a classic for steaks. If you substitute orange juice (preferably from a blood orange) for lemon juice, you'll have Sauce Maltaise, which is delicious with vegetables.

1. Melt the butter in a saucepan over very low heat. While the butter is melting, blend all the other ingredients except the salt in a blender or food processor.

2. With the blender running on medium speed, slowly add the butter, a little at a time. Return the sauce to a low heat and whisk until thickened. Add the salt and serve immediately.

PER SERVING (1 OUNCE): Calories: 161 | Fat: 17 g | Protein: 2 g | Sodium: 60 mg | Fiber: 0 g | Carbohydrates: 0 g | Sugar: 0 g | GI: Zero

Mango Salsa

This salsa is excellent with shrimp, crab legs, or fruit.
Avoid using frozen mango since it tends to be mushy when thawed.

INGREDIENTS | MAKES 1 CUP

1 mango, peeled and diced

¼ cup minced sweet onion

2 teaspoons cider vinegar

2 jalapeños, cored, seeded, and minced

Juice of ½ lime

2 tablespoons finely chopped cilantro or parsley

Salt to taste

Pulse all ingredients in the food processor or blender. Turn the mixture into a bowl, chill, and serve.

> **PER SERVING (1 OUNCE):** Calories: 209 | Fat: 0 g | Protein: 2 g | Sodium: 108 mg | Fiber: 2 g | Carbohydrates: 54 g | Sugar: 8 g | GI: Low

Sesame Mayonnaise

This dressing is great on beef, turkey, or chicken burgers.

INGREDIENTS | SERVES 8

2 large eggs

2 tablespoons lemon juice

1 teaspoon mustard powder

2 tablespoons tahini paste

1½ cups olive oil

1. Combine eggs, lemon juice, mustard powder, and tahini paste in a food processor, and pulse until blended.

2. Slowly drizzle the olive oil into the egg mixture and continue to pulse until completely blended.

> **PER SERVING:** Calories: 402 | Fat: 44 g | Protein: 2 g | Sodium: 20 mg | Fiber: 0.5 g | Carbohydrates: 1 g | Sugar: 0 g | GI: Zero

CHAPTER 18

Stews and Soups

Carrot Lemon Soup

This is a great anytime soup and can be served either hot or cold.

2 pounds carrots

2 large yellow onions

2 cloves garlic

3 tablespoons olive oil

6 cups low-sodium chicken broth or Basic Vegetable Stock (see recipe in this chapter)

1 teaspoon minced fresh ginger

1 fresh lemon, juice and zest

Freshly cracked black pepper to taste

3 fresh scallions, for garnish

1. Peel and dice the carrots and onions. Mince the garlic.

2. Heat the oil in a large stockpot over medium heat and lightly sauté the carrots, onions, and garlic for 3–5 minutes.

3. Add the broth/stock and simmer for approximately 1 hour. Add the ginger, lemon juice, and zest. Season with pepper.

4. Chill and serve with finely chopped scallions as garnish.

PER SERVING: Calories: 153 | Fat: 7 g | Protein: 3 g | Sodium: 62 mg | Fiber: 5 g | Carbohydrates: 16 g | Sugar: 5 g | GI: Moderate

Lemon Know-How

The thought of lemons may make your cheeks pucker, but they're well worth the powerful dose of cold-fighting vitamin C. The average lemon contains approximately 3 tablespoons of juice. Allow lemons to come to room temperature before squeezing to maximize the amount of juice extracted.

Pumpkin Soup

This is a perfect autumn soup to celebrate the harvest season. If you're short on time or pumpkins are out of season, substitute 1 (15-ounce) can of puréed pumpkin for the fresh pumpkin.

INGREDIENTS | SERVES 6

2 cups large-diced fresh sugar pumpkin, seeds reserved separately

Salt to taste

3 leeks, sliced

1½ teaspoons minced fresh ginger

1 tablespoon olive oil

½ teaspoon grated fresh lemon zest

1 teaspoon fresh lemon juice

2 quarts low-sodium vegetable stock or Basic Vegetable Stock (see recipe in this chapter)

½ teaspoon sea salt

Freshly ground black pepper to taste

1 tablespoon extra-virgin olive oil, for drizzling

Zesting

If you don't have a zester, you can still easily make lemon zest. Simply use your cheese grater, but be careful to grate only the rind and not the white pith, which tends to be bitter.

1. Preheat the oven to 375°F.

2. Clean the pumpkin seeds thoroughly, place them on a baking sheet, and sprinkle with salt. Roast for approximately 5–8 minutes, until light golden.

3. Place the diced pumpkin in a baking dish with the leeks, ginger, and olive oil; roast for 45 minutes–1 hour, until cooked al dente.

4. Transfer the cooked pumpkin to a large stockpot and add the zest, juice, stock, salt and pepper; place over low heat and let simmer for 30–45 minutes.

5. To serve, ladle into serving bowls. Drizzle with extra-virgin olive oil and sprinkle with toasted pumpkin seeds.

PER SERVING: Calories: 100 | Fat: 4 g | Protein: 3 g | Sodium: 62 mg | Fiber: 1.5 g | Carbohydrates: 10 g | Sugar: 3 g | GI: Moderate

Butternut Squash Soup

This soup is a scrumptious treat on a cool fall day.
Warm family and friends with a delightful blend of aroma and flavor.

INGREDIENTS | SERVES 4

1 tablespoon olive oil

1 medium onion, peeled and chopped

1 pound butternut squash, peeled, seeded, and chopped

½ cup flax meal

4 cups low-sodium chicken broth or homemade stock

1 cup almond milk

½ teaspoon ground cinnamon

¼ teaspoon ground cloves

¼ teaspoon ground nutmeg

1. In a soup pot or Dutch oven, heat olive oil on medium-high. Sauté the onion and butternut squash in oil for 5 minutes.

2. Add the flax meal and chicken broth/stock, and increase heat to high.

3. Bring to a boil, then turn to low, and simmer for 45 minutes.

4. In batches, purée the squash mixture in a blender or food processor and return to the pot.

5. Stir in the almond milk, cinnamon, cloves, and nutmeg.

PER SERVING: Calories: 182 | Fat: 9 g | Protein: 8.5 g | Sodium: 495 mg | Fiber: 5.5 g | Carbohydrates: 20 g | Sugar: 9 g | GI: Moderate

Cream of Cauliflower Soup

Cauliflower is a fantastic vegetable. Blended cauliflower can be used as a thickener in recipes that normally call for potatoes or root vegetables. Best of all, cauliflower won't spike your insulin levels.

INGREDIENTS | SERVES 4

1 large head cauliflower, chopped
3 stalks celery, chopped
1 medium carrot, peeled and chopped
2 cloves garlic, minced
1 onion, peeled and chopped
2 teaspoons ground cumin
½ teaspoon freshly ground black pepper
1 tablespoon chopped parsley
¼ teaspoon dill

1. In a soup pot or Dutch oven, combine the cauliflower, celery, carrot, garlic, onions, cumin, and pepper.

2. Add enough water to cover the ingredients in the pot. Bring to a boil over high.

3. Reduce heat to low. Simmer about 8 minutes or until the vegetables are tender.

4. Stir in the parsley and dill before serving.

PER SERVING: Calories: 56 | Fat: 0.5 g | Protein: 3 g | Sodium: 83 mg | Fiber: 5 g | Carbohydrates: 10 g | Sugar: 2 g | GI: Very low

Basic Chicken Soup

The major advantage of this soup is that it will be much lower in sodium than canned chicken soups. The only limit is your imagination. Each time you make it, substitute different vegetables and seasonings to tantalize your taste buds.

INGREDIENTS | SERVES 6

5–6 pounds chicken (including giblets)
2 medium carrots
2 stalks celery
4 large yellow onions
¼ bunch parsley, chopped
12 cups water
Freshly cracked black pepper to taste
Kosher salt to taste

1. Clean, trim, and quarter the chicken. Peel and chop all the vegetables.

2. Place the chicken and giblets in a stockpot, add the water, and bring to a boil. Reduce the heat to a simmer and skim off all foam.

3. Add all the remaining ingredients and simmer uncovered for about 3 hours.

4. Remove the chicken and giblets from the stockpot; discard the giblets. Remove the meat from the bones, discard the bones, and return the meat to the broth; serve.

PER SERVING: Calories: 183 | Fat: 8 g | Protein: 16 g | Sodium: 84 mg | Fiber: 1.5 g | Carbohydrates: 5.5 g | Sugar: 2 g | GI: Low

Basic Vegetable Stock

Another great broth that is packed with health-promoting phytochemicals.
Try adding mushrooms for additional flavor.

INGREDIENTS | MAKES 1 GALLON

2 pounds yellow onions
1 pound carrots
1 pound celery
1 bunch fresh parsley stems
1½ gallons water
4 stems fresh thyme
2 bay leaves (fresh or dried)
10–20 peppercorns

Homemade Stocks

Homemade stocks give a special quality to any dish. Not only will the flavor of home-made stocks be better than that of pur-chased bases, but you will have added your own personal touch to the meal. Always cook them uncovered, as covering will cause them to become cloudy.

1. Peel and roughly chop the onions and carrots. Roughly chop the celery (stalks only; no leaves) and the fresh parsley stems.

2. Put the vegetables and water in a stockpot over medium heat; bring to a simmer and cook, uncovered, for 1½ hours.

3. Add the herbs and peppercorns, and continue to sim-mer, uncovered, for 45 minutes. Adjust seasonings to taste as necessary.

4. Remove from heat and cool by submerging the pot in a bath of ice and water. Place in freezer-safe containers and store in the freezer until ready to use. Remove the bay leaves before serving.

PER SERVING (1 CUP): Calories: 22 | Fat: 0 g | Protein: 0 g | Sodium: 31 mg | Fiber: 0 g | Carbohydrates: 5.3 g | Sugar: 2 g | GI: Low

Simple Ground Turkey and Vegetable Soup

This soup is easy to throw together with ingredients from the pantry.

INGREDIENTS | SERVES 6

1 tablespoon olive oil

1 pound ground turkey

1 medium onion, peeled and diced

2 cloves garlic, minced

1 (16-ounce) package frozen mixed vegetables

4 cups gluten-free chicken broth or homemade stock

½ teaspoon freshly ground black pepper

½ teaspoon salt

1. In a large skillet on medium, heat the olive oil until sizzling. Cook the ground turkey until browned, about 5–6 minutes, stirring to break up the meat. Add the meat to a greased 4-quart slow cooker. Sauté the onion and garlic until softened, about 3–5 minutes. Add to the slow cooker.

2. Add the remaining ingredients. Cover and cook on high for 4 hours or on low for 8 hours. Serve hot.

PER SERVING: Calories: 254 | Fat: 11.5 g | Protein: 19 g | Sodium: 1001 mg | Fiber: 3.5 g | Carbohydrates: 20 g | Sugar: 1 g | GI: Very low

Broccoli Soup with Cheese

There is a lot to love about broccoli soup. Both nourishing and full of fiber, it can be enriched with cream or heated up with spicy pepper jack cheese.

INGREDIENTS | SERVES 4

¼ cup olive oil

1 medium sweet onion, peeled and chopped

2 cloves garlic, chopped

1 large baking potato, peeled and chopped

1 large bunch organic broccoli, coarsely chopped

½ cup dry white wine

3 cups chicken broth or homemade stock

Salt and pepper to taste

Pinch ground nutmeg

4 heaping tablespoons grated extra-sharp Cheddar

1. Heat the olive oil in a large soup kettle. Sauté the onion, garlic, and potato over medium heat until softened slightly. Add the broccoli, liquids, and seasonings.

2. Cover the soup and simmer over low heat for 45 minutes.

3. Cool slightly. Purée in the blender. Reheat and place in bowls.

4. Spoon the cheese over the hot soup to serve.

PER SERVING: Calories: 297 | Fat: 19 g | Protein: 8 g | Sodium: 623 mg | Fiber: 3 g | Carbohydrates: 22 g | Sugar: 2 g | GI: Very low

Mediterranean Seafood Soup

This quick and easy soup will give you a taste of the Mediterranean.

INGREDIENTS | SERVES 2

2 tablespoons olive oil

½ cup chopped sweet onion

2 cloves garlic, chopped

½ bulb fennel, chopped

½ cup dry white wine

1 cup clam broth

2 cups chopped tomatoes

6 littleneck clams, tightly closed

6 mussels, tightly closed

8 raw shrimp, jumbo, peeled and deveined

1 teaspoon dried basil, or 5 leaves fresh basil, torn

Salt and red pepper flakes to taste

1. In a Dutch oven or stockpot, heat the oil over medium-high heat, and add the onion, garlic, and fennel. After 10 minutes, stir in the wine and clam broth and add the tomatoes. Bring to a boil.

2. Drop the clams into the boiling liquid. When the clams start to open, add the mussels. When the mussels start to open, add the shrimp, basil, salt, and pepper flakes. Serve when the shrimp turns pink.

PER SERVING: Calories: 450 | Fat: 18 g | Protein: 48 g | Sodium: 1355 mg | Fiber: 1 g | Carbohydrates: 19 g | Sugar: 2 g | GI: Very low

Littleneck Clams

Littleneck clams are the smallest variety of hard-shell clams and can be found on the northeastern and northwestern coasts of the United States. They have a sweet taste and are delicious steamed and dipped in melted butter, battered and fried, or baked.

Savory Fish Stew

This stew is fresh and easy to make and has a whole lot of flavor.
The recipe calls for halibut, but just about any meaty whitefish will do.

INGREDIENTS | SERVES 6

1 tablespoon olive oil

1 medium onion, peeled and finely chopped

½ cup dry white wine

3 large tomatoes, chopped

2 cups low-sodium chicken broth or homemade stock

8 ounces clam juice

3 cups fresh spinach

1 pound halibut fillets, cut into 1" pieces

White pepper to taste

1 tablespoon chopped fresh cilantro

1. Place a large frying pan over medium heat. Add the oil to the pan and sauté the onions for 2–3 minutes. Add wine to deglaze the pan. Scrape the pan to loosen the small bits of onion.

2. Add the tomatoes and cook for 3–4 minutes; then add the broth/stock and clam juice to the pan. Stir in the spinach and allow it to wilt while continuing to stir.

3. Season the fish with pepper, place the fish in the pan, and cook for 5–6 minutes until opaque. Mix in the cilantro before serving.

PER SERVING: Calories: 157 | Fat: 7 g | Protein: 19 g | Sodium: 321 mg | Fiber: 2 g | Carbohydrates: 7 g | Sugar: 1 g | GI: Very low

Thai Chicken Stew with Vegetables in Coconut Cream

*Asian flavorings can provide so many minimal, yet wonderful, additions
to rather ordinary foods. This chicken stew is spicy and tastes very rich.
It is loaded with vegetables that reduce the GI value of this dish. Try it served over rice.*

INGREDIENTS | SERVES 4

2 cloves garlic, minced

1 (1") piece fresh ginger, peeled and minced

2 tablespoons peanut oil

2 medium carrots, peeled and shredded

1 cup canned coconut cream

1 cup gluten-free chicken broth or homemade stock

2 cups shredded napa cabbage

4 (5-ounce) boneless, skinless (optional) chicken breasts, cut into bite-size pieces

¼ cup gluten-free soy sauce

2 tablespoons fish sauce

1 teaspoon Thai chili paste (red or green) or red hot-pepper sauce

1 tablespoon sesame oil

½ cup chopped scallion (green part only)

¼ cup chopped cilantro

1. In a large Dutch oven or stockpot, sauté the garlic and ginger in the peanut oil over medium-high heat for 3–5 minutes. Add the carrots, coconut cream, and chicken broth, and simmer for 10 minutes. Add the cabbage, chicken, soy sauce, and fish sauce.

2. Whisk in the chili paste. Stir in the sesame oil, scallions, and cilantro. Simmer for 20 minutes.

PER SERVING: Calories: 540 | Fat: 35 g | Protein: 55 g | Sodium: 778 mg | Fiber: 2 g | Carbohydrates: 16 g | Sugar: 3 g | GI: Low

Coconut Cream, Coconut Milk, Coconut Juice

Contrary to popular belief, coconut milk is not the liquid found inside a whole coconut (that is called coconut water or coconut juice). Coconut milk is made by mixing water with shredded coconut and then squeezing the mixture through cheesecloth to filter out the coconut pieces. Coconut cream is the same as coconut milk, but it is made with less water and more coconut.

Egg Drop Soup with Lemon

This is a lovely spicy version of the Chinese staple, made with a variety of Asian sauces. Asian fish sauce is a liquid made from salted fish that is used instead of salt in many Asian recipes. Hoisin sauce is made from crushed soybeans and garlic, has a sweet and spicy flavor, and is a rich brown color.

INGREDIENTS | SERVES 2

1 tablespoon peanut oil

1 clove garlic, minced

2 cups gluten-free chicken broth or homemade stock

Juice of ½ lemon

1 tablespoon gluten-free hoisin sauce

1 teaspoon gluten-free soy sauce

1 teaspoon fish sauce

½ teaspoon chili oil, or to taste

1 (1") piece fresh ginger, peeled and minced

2 eggs

1. Heat the peanut oil in a large saucepan. Sauté the garlic over medium heat until softened, about 5 minutes.

2. Add the chicken broth/stock, lemon juice, hoisin sauce, soy sauce, fish sauce, chili oil, and ginger. Stir and cover. Cook over low heat for 20 minutes.

3. Just before serving, whisk the eggs with a fork. Add to the boiling soup and continue to whisk until the eggs form thin strands.

PER SERVING: Calories: 158 | Fat: 13 g | Protein: 5 g | Sodium: 599 mg | Fiber: 0 g | Carbohydrates: 2 g | Sugar: 2 g | GI: Very low

CHAPTER 19

Salads

Greek Salad

Olives are a rich source of oleic acid, a heart-healthy monounsaturated fat. While various types of olives are commonly used in Mediterranean dishes, Greek salads often feature kalamata olives.

INGREDIENTS | SERVES 4

4 cups chopped romaine lettuce

1 large tomato, seeds removed and chopped

1 small cucumber, sliced

1 medium organic green bell pepper, seeded and cut into rings

½ cup feta cheese

¼ cup red wine vinegar

Juice of 1 lemon

1 tablespoon Italian seasoning

Salt and pepper to taste

¼ cup extra-virgin olive oil

2 teaspoons capers

16 kalamata olives

1. Place the lettuce, tomato, cucumber, bell pepper, and feta in a large bowl.

2. To make the dressing, whisk the vinegar, lemon juice, Italian seasoning, salt, and pepper in a small bowl; mix in the olive oil.

3. Coat the vegetables with the dressing.

4. Place the salad on plates. Top with capers and olives.

PER SERVING: Calories: 228 | Fat: 7 g | Protein: 5 g | Sodium: 799 mg | Fiber: 3 g | Carbohydrates: 20 g | Sugar: 1 g | GI: Low

Feta Is "Betta"

Greek shepherds have been making feta cheese for centuries. Originally made from goat's or sheep's milk, feta today is produced from pasteurized cow's milk. In Greece, feta cheese is served in restaurants and homes as a garnish on various types of fresh salads.

Cucumber Salad with Yogurt and Dill

This cool and refreshing salad pairs well with a spicy grilled meat for a relaxing summer barbecue.

INGREDIENTS | SERVES 2

2 large cucumbers

1 cup plain yogurt

1 tablespoon apple cider vinegar

2 tablespoons finely chopped fresh dill

Salt and pepper to taste

1. Wash and peel the cucumbers; chop into ¼"-thick slices.

2. In a medium bowl, combine the cucumber with the yogurt, vinegar, dill, salt, and pepper.

3. Serve chilled.

PER SERVING: Calories: 109 | Fat: 2 g | Protein: 8 g | Sodium: 625 mg | Fiber: 2 g | Carbohydrates: 14 g | Sugar: 5 g | GI: Low

Making a Cucumber Raita

This recipe may be modified to make raita, an Indian cuisine condiment. Chop the cucumber into ¼" cubes. Substitute 2 tablespoons chopped mint leaves for the dill; add a minced garlic clove and cayenne pepper to taste.

Mediterranean Tomato Salad

Use juicy tomatoes for this recipe, such as heirloom or beefsteak.
You can substitute orange bell pepper for the yellow if needed.

INGREDIENTS | SERVES 4

2 cups sliced tomatoes

1 cup peeled and chopped cucumber

⅓ cup diced organic yellow bell pepper

¼ cup sliced radishes

¼ cup chopped flat-leaf parsley

1 garlic clove, finely minced

1 tablespoon lemon juice

3 tablespoons extra-virgin olive oil

Salt and pepper to taste

2 cups torn organic baby spinach leaves

1. Toss the tomatoes, cucumbers, bell pepper, radishes, and parsley in a large salad bowl.

2. Sprinkle the garlic, lemon juice, and oil over the salad. Toss to coat. Salt and pepper to taste. Split the spinach among four plates and top with the salad. Serve immediately.

PER SERVING: Calories: 131 | Fat: 10 g | Protein: 2.5 g | Sodium: 71 mg | Fiber: 2.5 g | Carbohydrates: 7 g | Sugar: 3 g | GI: Low

Baby Vegetable Salad

Use the smallest vegetables available for this salad. Garnish with spicy prosciutto and sweet fennel.

INGREDIENTS | SERVES 4

¼ cup olive oil

2 cloves garlic, minced

12 tiny fresh white onions, peeled

1 pound tiny haricots verts (French green beans)

1 bulb fennel, trimmed and thinly sliced

5 ounces small white button mushrooms

8 baby carrots

¼ cup apple cider vinegar

¼ cup shredded fresh basil

¼ cup shredded fresh parsley

Salt and pepper to taste

½ cup stemmed, loosely packed watercress

1 head organic lettuce, shredded

½ pound currant or grape tomatoes

½ pound Black Forest ham, chopped

1. In a large sauté pan, heat the olive oil over medium-low and sauté the garlic, onions, haricots verts, fennel, mushrooms, and carrots until the haricots verts and carrots are crisp-tender, about 4–5 minutes.

2. Stir in the apple cider vinegar, basil, and parsley. Sprinkle with salt and pepper to taste.

3. When the vegetables are at room temperature, arrange the watercress and lettuce on serving plates and spoon on the vegetables. Add tomatoes. Sprinkle with the ham and serve.

PER SERVING: Calories: 346 | Fat: 20 g | Protein: 19 g | Sodium: 634 mg | Fiber: 5 g | Carbohydrates: 18 g | Sugar: 3 g | GI: Low

Arugula and Fennel Salad with Pomegranate

Pomegranates pack a high dose of beneficial health-promoting antioxidants. They are in peak season October through January; you can also substitute dried cranberries.

INGREDIENTS | SERVES 4

2 large navel oranges

1 pomegranate

4 cups organic arugula

1 cup thinly sliced fennel

4 tablespoons olive oil

Salt and pepper to taste

Fennel Facts

Fennel, a crunchy and slightly sweet vegetable, is a popular Mediterranean ingredient. Fennel has a white or greenish-white bulb and long stalks with feathery green leaves stemming from the top. Fennel is closely related to cilantro, dill, carrots, and parsley.

1. Cut the tops and bottoms off the oranges and then cut away the remaining peel. Slice each orange into 10–12 small pieces.

2. Remove the seeds from the pomegranate.

3. Place the arugula, orange pieces, pomegranate seeds, and fennel slices into a large bowl.

4. Coat the salad with olive oil and season with salt and pepper as desired.

PER SERVING: Calories: 224 | Fat: 15 g | Protein: 3 g | Sodium: 609 mg | Carbohydrates: 24 g | Sugar: 15 g | GI: Low

Fig and Parmesan Curl Salad

This mixture may sound a bit different, and it is! In addition to being unique, it is also delicious.

INGREDIENTS | SERVES 2

4 fresh figs, cut into halves, or 4 dried figs, plumped in 1 cup boiling water and soaked for ½ hour

2 cups stemmed fresh organic baby spinach

¼ cup olive oil

Juice of ½ lemon

2 tablespoons balsamic vinegar

1 teaspoon honey

1 teaspoon dark brown mustard

Salt and pepper to taste

4 large curls Parmesan cheese

1. When the figs (if dried) are softened, prepare the spinach and arrange on serving dishes.

2. In a bowl, whisk the olive oil, lemon juice, balsamic vinegar, honey, mustard, salt, and pepper. Place Parmesan curls over the figs and spinach; drizzle with the dressing.

PER SERVING: Calories: 284 | Fat: 16 g | Protein: 10 g | Sodium: 1368 mg | Carbohydrates: 30 g | Sugar: 22 g | GI: Low

Orange Salad

This bright, citrusy salad is a perfect fall side dish.

INGREDIENTS | SERVES 4

3 cups cubed butternut squash, drizzled with olive oil and roasted

2 medium carrots, peeled and shredded

2 cups diced papaya

2 tablespoons shredded fresh ginger

Juice of 1 lime

1 tablespoon honey, or to taste

1 tablespoon olive oil

½ teaspoon sea salt

Freshly ground black pepper to taste

1. Combine the squash, carrots, and papaya in a large salad bowl. Set aside.

2. In a small bowl, mix the ginger, lime juice, honey, olive oil, salt, and pepper until well combined.

3. Toss the dressing with the salad ingredients and serve.

PER SERVING: Calories: 142 | Fat: 3.5 g | Protein: 2 g | Sodium: 621 mg | Fiber: 5 g | Carbohydrates: 29 g | Sugar: 13 g | GI: Moderate

Root Vegetable Salad

This root salad has a nice texture and color. It will go well with any traditional fall or winter dish and will make your home smell like a holiday meal.

INGREDIENTS | SERVES 4

1 rutabaga, peeled and cubed
1 turnip, peeled and cubed
6 parsnips, peeled and cubed
3 tablespoons olive oil
1 tablespoon ground cinnamon
3 cloves garlic, chopped
1 tablespoon ground ginger
1 teaspoon freshly ground black pepper

Root Vegetables

These underground vegetables are recommended as they are high in vitamin A and are a nice form of carbohydrate fuel, particularly after exercising.

1. Preheat the oven to 400°F.

2. Place the rutabaga, turnip, and parsnips in a roasting pan and drizzle with olive oil.

3. Sprinkle them with the cinnamon, garlic, ginger, and pepper.

4. Toss them in the pan to coat and roast for 40–50 minutes or until a toothpick slides easily through the vegetables.

PER SERVING: Calories: 247 | Fat: 11 g | Protein: 4 g | Sodium: 79 mg | Fiber: 11 g | Carbohydrates: 36 g | Sugar: 15 g | GI: Moderate

Pineapple Onion Salad

This sweet and tangy recipe does not keep well, so make sure to throw it together right before eating. If you prefer a little more zing, add another tablespoon of lime juice and a sprinkle of cayenne pepper.

INGREDIENTS | SERVES 4

1 cup cubed fresh pineapple
½ cup chopped red onion
3 cups mixed organic baby greens
1 tablespoon lime juice

1. Place the pineapple chunks in a large salad bowl. Mix the onions and baby greens into the pineapple.

2. Sprinkle the salad lightly with lime juice. Toss to coat and serve immediately.

PER SERVING: Calories: 28 | Fat: 0 g | Protein: 0 g | Sodium: 1 mg | Fiber: 1 g | Carbohydrates: 5.5 g | Sugar: 4 g | GI: Low

Kale and Sea Vegetables with Orange-Sesame Dressing

This salad is a great appetizer for an Asian-themed meal.

INGREDIENTS | SERVES 4

¼ cup wakame seaweed

½ cup sea lettuce

3 cups organic kale

½ teaspoon lemon juice

¼ cup fresh squeezed orange juice

6 tablespoons plus 1 teaspoon sesame seeds

1 tablespoon kelp powder

Sea Vegetables

Sea vegetables are among the most nutritious and mineral-rich foods on earth. Ocean water contains all the mineral elements known to humans. For example, both kelp and dulse, different types of seaweed, are excellent sources of iodine, which is an essential nutrient missing in most diets. Sea vegetables are dried and should be reconstituted by soaking them in water before eating.

1. Soak the wakame and sea lettuce in water for 30 minutes. Rinse the vegetables and discard the water.

2. Remove the stems from the kale. Roll the kale leaves and chop them into small pieces.

3. Sprinkle the lemon juice onto the kale and massage it by hand to create a wilting effect.

4. Place the orange juice, 6 tablespoons of sesame seeds, and kelp powder into a blender and blend until smooth.

5. Toss the dressing with the kale and sea vegetables in a large bowl until well covered. Sprinkle the remaining sesame seeds on top.

PER SERVING: Calories: 90 | Fat: 5 g | Protein: 4 g | Sodium: 64 mg | Fiber: 3 g | Carbohydrates: 9 g | Sugar: 2 g | GI: Very low

Red Pepper and Fennel Salad

Fennel has a fantastic licorice flavor that blends nicely with nuts.
The red pepper adds a flash of color and a bit of sweetness to the mix.

INGREDIENTS | SERVES 2

⅓ cup pine nuts, toasted

3 tablespoons sesame seeds, toasted

2 tablespoons olive oil

1 medium organic red bell pepper, seeded and halved

6 leaves organic romaine lettuce, shredded

½ bulb fennel, diced

1 tablespoon walnut oil

Juice from 1 lime

Freshly ground black pepper to taste

Walnut Oil

Walnut oil cannot withstand high heat, so it's best to add it to food that has been cooked or is served raw, such as a salad. If you choose to cook with walnut oil, use a lower flame to avoid burning it.

1. Preheat the broiler.

2. In a medium skillet, sauté the pine nuts and sesame seeds in olive oil over medium heat for 5 minutes.

3. Grill the pepper under the broiler until the skin is blackened and the flesh has softened slightly, about 5–8 minutes.

4. Place the pepper halves in a paper bag to cool slightly. When cool enough to handle, remove the skin and slice the pepper into strips.

5. Combine the red pepper slices, lettuce, and fennel in a large salad bowl.

6. Add the walnut oil, lime juice, and black pepper to taste. Mix the dressing well with the salad. Add the nut mixture and serve.

PER SERVING: Calories: 456 | Fat: 43 g | Protein: 7 g | Sodium: 37 mg | Fiber: 6 g | Carbohydrates: 17 g | Sugar: 5 g | GI: Low

Broccoli, Pine Nut, and Apple Salad

This quick little salad will tide you over to your next meal. The broccoli and apple taste great together and the toasted pine nuts add a bit of a crunch.

INGREDIENTS | SERVES 2

4 tablespoons olive oil
¾ cup pine nuts
2 cups organic broccoli florets
2 cups diced organic green apples
Juice of 1 lemon

1. Heat the olive oil in a small frying pan and sauté the pine nuts over medium heat until golden brown, about 3–4 minutes.

2. Mix the broccoli and apples in a medium bowl. Add the pine nuts and toss.

3. Squeeze the lemon juice over the salad and serve.

PER SERVING: Calories: 621 | Fat: 53 g | Protein: 15 g | Sodium: 34 mg | Fiber: 7 g | Carbohydrates: 31 g | Sugar: 9 g | GI: Low

CHAPTER 20

Vegetables

Roasted Green Beans with Pine Nuts

Dress up your everyday green beans with toasted pine nuts, crispy prosciutto, and fresh sage.

INGREDIENTS | SERVES 6

2 pounds organic green beans, trimmed

2 ounces prosciutto or bacon, thinly sliced

2 teaspoons olive oil

4 cloves garlic, minced

2 teaspoons fresh sage, minced

¼ teaspoon salt, divided

Freshly ground black pepper to taste

¼ cup pine nuts, toasted

1 teaspoon lemon zest

Toasting Nuts and Seeds

Place nuts or seeds in a dry skillet over medium-low heat and cook for 3–5 minutes. Nuts will have a nutty scent and will be slightly browned.

1. Boil water in a large pot. Add the green beans to the pot and simmer until they are crisp-tender, about 4 minutes. Drain the green beans.

2. Place a large frying pan over medium heat. Add the prosciutto and cook, stirring, until crisp, about 3–4 minutes. Transfer the prosciutto to a paper towel to absorb any excess oil.

3. Add the olive oil to the large pan and return to medium heat. Add the green beans, garlic, sage, ⅛ teaspoon salt, and pepper to the pan. Cook until the green beans begin to brown slightly, about 6–8 minutes.

4. Add in the pine nuts, lemon zest, and prosciutto; season with the remaining salt and additional pepper.

PER SERVING: Calories: 99 | Fat: 5 g | Protein: 5 g | Sodium: 449 mg | Fiber: 5 g | Carbohydrates: 10 g | Sugar: 3 g | GI: Low

Spring Greens with Berries

The acid in the lime juice breaks down the fat in the olive oil to make a flavorful dressing.

INGREDIENTS | SERVES 2

1 jalapeño
4 tablespoons lime juice
4 tablespoons olive oil
¼ teaspoon ground cumin
4 cups mixed organic baby greens
2 cups fresh organic blackberries or raspberries
¼ cup thinly sliced red onion

1. Slice the jalapeño and remove the seeds and stem. Mince the pepper flesh.

2. Place the lime juice, olive oil, cumin, and 2 teaspoons of the minced jalapeño into a blender and blend until smooth.

3. Toss the dressing with the greens, berries, and onions and serve as a side salad.

PER SERVING: Calories: 363 | Fat: 28 g | Protein: 5.5 g | Sodium: 242 mg | Fiber: 9.5 g | Carbohydrates: 21 g | Sugar: 6 g | GI: Low

Marinated Baby Artichoke Hearts

Here's where frozen artichoke hearts work perfectly! They save you the time and energy of cutting out the choke and removing the leaves of fresh artichokes, and they are delicious marinated.

INGREDIENTS | SERVES 4

2 (9- or 10-ounce) boxes frozen artichoke hearts
½ cup apple cider vinegar
¼ cup olive oil
1 teaspoon Dijon-style mustard
½ teaspoon ground coriander seeds
Salt and pepper to taste

1. Thaw and cook the artichokes according to package directions. Drain.

2. Whisk the rest of the ingredients in a bowl large enough to hold the artichokes. Add the warm artichokes and cover with the dressing. Cover and marinate for 2–4 hours. Serve as an antipasto.

PER SERVING: Calories: 142 | Fat: 15 g | Protein: 1 g | Sodium: 430 mg | Fiber: 6 g | Carbohydrates: 4 g | Sugar: 1 g | GI: Very low

Cinnamon-Toasted Butternut Squash

This side dish or snack is a great fall dish. It smells amazing and will give you the carbohydrate boost your glycogen storage needs.

INGREDIENTS | SERVES 4

3 cups cubed butternut squash
1 tablespoon ground cinnamon
1 teaspoon ground nutmeg

1. Preheat the oven to 350°F.

2. Place the squash in a 9" × 11" baking dish. Sprinkle with the cinnamon and nutmeg.

3. Bake for 30 minutes or until tender and slightly brown.

PER SERVING: Calories: 93 | Fat: 0 g | Protein: 1 g | Sodium: 7 mg | Fiber: 3 g | Carbohydrates: 24 g | Sugar: 12 g | GI: Moderate

Broccoli Rabe with Lemon and Cheese

Broccoli rabe is somewhat bitter and has a real snap to its flavor. It is wonderful when poached in boiling water and then sautéed in oil with a bit of garlic and lemon juice. Serve this recipe over rice or pasta, or on its own.

INGREDIENTS | SERVES 4

1 quart water
1 teaspoon salt
½ cup loosely packed organic broccoli rabe, ends trimmed
2 tablespoons olive oil
2 cloves garlic, chopped
1 tablespoon lemon juice
Salt and pepper to taste
2 tablespoons grated Parmesan

1. In a large saucepan, bring the water to a boil; add the salt and broccoli rabe. Reduce heat and simmer on low for 6–8 minutes. Drain and shock under cold water and dry on paper towels.

2. In a medium frying pan, heat the olive oil on medium-low and sauté the garlic for 5 minutes. Cut the broccoli rabe stems in 2" pieces and add to the garlic and olive oil. Sprinkle with the lemon juice, salt, and pepper. Serve with Parmesan.

PER SERVING: Calories: 81 | Fat: 8 g | Protein: 2 g | Sodium: 1238 mg | Fiber: 1 g | Carbohydrates: 2 g | Sugar: 0 g | GI: Zero

Roasted Asparagus

Use thicker asparagus to withstand the heat of the grill.
Be sure to remove the woody end of the stalks first.

INGREDIENTS | SERVES 6

2 bunches asparagus
1 tablespoon extra-virgin olive oil
Lemon juice to taste (optional)
Freshly cracked black pepper to taste

Asparagus

Asparagus is low in calories and sodium, and offers numerous vitamins and minerals, most notably folate and potassium. The stalks also offer a blast of inflammation-fighting antioxidants.

Preheat the grill to medium. Toss the asparagus in the oil, drain it on a rack, and season with lemon juice and pepper. Grill the asparagus 1–2 minutes on each side (cook to desired doneness). Serve immediately.

PER SERVING: Calories: 30 | Fat: 2 g | Protein: 1 g | Sodium: 1 mg | Fiber: 1 g | Carbohydrates: 2 g | Sugar: 1 g | GI: Very low

Mediterranean Green Beans

This simple recipe can be served hot or at room temperature. Add any leftovers to your salads.

INGREDIENTS | SERVES 4

1 pound fresh organic green beans, ends trimmed, cut into 1" pieces
2 teaspoons minced fresh rosemary
1 teaspoon lemon zest
1 tablespoon olive oil
Freshly cracked black pepper to taste

Taking Care of Your Produce

Store unwashed fresh green beans in a reusable bag in the refrigerator. When you are ready to use them, wash the beans under cold running water.

1. Fill a medium saucepan with cold salted water and bring the water to a boil on high. Add the beans and cook until they are a vibrant green, about 4 minutes.

2. Drain the beans and transfer to a large bowl. Add the remaining ingredients and toss to coat evenly. Serve warm or at room temperature.

PER SERVING: Calories: 70 | Fat: 3.5 g | Protein: 2 g | Sodium: 22 mg | Fiber: 3.5 g | Carbohydrates: 9 g | Sugar: 2 g

Chipotle-Lime Mashed Sweet Potatoes

Sweet potatoes are a great food for after a workout. This dish will be a favorite at any family table.

INGREDIENTS | SERVES 10

3 pounds sweet potatoes
1½ tablespoons coconut oil
1¼ teaspoons chipotle powder
Juice from ½ large lime

Alternatives to Sweet Potatoes

If you don't like sweet potatoes, you can easily substitute some lower-glycemic-load vegetables such as rutabagas, turnips, or beets. Additionally, cauliflower makes a great fake "mashed potato" substitute.

1. Peel the sweet potatoes and cut them into cubes.

2. Steam the cubes until soft, approximately 5–8 minutes. Transfer them to a large bowl.

3. In a small saucepan, heat the coconut oil and whisk in the chipotle powder and lime juice.

4. Pour the mixture into the bowl with the sweet potato cubes and mash them with a fork or potato masher. Serve immediately.

PER SERVING: Calories: 135 | Fat: 2 g | Protein: 2.5 g | Sodium: 75 mg | Fiber: 4 g | Carbohydrates: 27 g | Sugar: 13 g | GI: Moderate

Slow-Cooked Collard Greens

This is a Southern staple that goes perfectly with barbecue chicken or ribs.

INGREDIENTS | SERVES 8

1 meaty smoked ham hock, rinsed

1 large carrot, peeled and chopped

1 large onion, peeled and chopped

1 (1-pound) package fresh chopped organic collard greens, with tough stems removed

1 teaspoon minced garlic

½ teaspoon crushed red pepper

¼ teaspoon freshly ground black pepper

6 cups gluten-free chicken broth or homemade stock

1 cup water

Make It Vegetarian

If you prefer, you can make these hearty greens without the ham hock. Simply leave it out, use vegetable broth instead of chicken broth, and add 1 (15-ounce) can of diced tomatoes (or your favorite salsa) and a few tablespoons of olive oil. Cook as directed and serve with the vegetable broth ladled over each serving.

1. Place the ham hock, carrots, and onions in a 6-quart slow cooker.

2. Add the collard greens. Sprinkle the greens with the garlic, red pepper, and black pepper.

3. Pour the broth/stock and water over the collard greens.

4. Cover and cook on low for 8 hours. To serve, remove the greens to a serving bowl. Remove the meat from the ham hock and discard the fat and bones. Chop the meat and add it to the greens. Ladle 1–2 cups broth over the greens.

PER SERVING: Calories: 193 | Fat: 7.5 g | Protein: 17.5 g | Sodium: 1580 mg | Fiber: 2.5 g | Carbohydrates: 14.5 g | Sugar: 1.2 g | GI: Low

Fingerling Potatoes with Herb Vinaigrette

Fingerling potatoes are small new potatoes. It's fun to use fingerling potatoes, because often they are small enough that they do not have to be chopped or diced. This dish is also delicious served cold as a potato salad.

INGREDIENTS | SERVES 4

2 pounds organic red or yellow fingerling potatoes, scrubbed

1 teaspoon salt

¼ cup lemon juice

⅓ cup extra-virgin olive oil

1 small shallot, minced (about 2 tablespoons)

1½ teaspoons minced fresh thyme leaves

1 tablespoon minced fresh basil leaves

1 tablespoon minced fresh oregano leaves

½ teaspoon Dijon mustard

1 teaspoon sugar

1. Place the potatoes in a medium pot and cover with cold water. Bring to a boil and add salt to the water. Cook the potatoes for 6–8 minutes until fork-tender.

2. Drain the potatoes and place them in a greased 4-quart slow cooker.

3. In a small bowl, whisk the lemon juice, olive oil, shallot, thyme, basil, oregano, mustard, and sugar. Drizzle the vinaigrette over the potatoes.

4. Cook on low for 4 hours or on high for 2 hours.

PER SERVING: Calories: 329 | Fat: 18 g | Protein: 4 g | Sodium: 615 mg | Fiber: 6 g | Carbohydrates: 39 g | Sugar: 4 g | GI: Moderate

Old-Fashioned Sweet Potato Hash Browns

These sweet potato hash browns are likely to become a family favorite. They are easy to make and packed with flavor your entire family will love.

INGREDIENTS | SERVES 6

3 tablespoons coconut oil

3 medium sweet potatoes, peeled and grated

1 tablespoon ground cinnamon

1. Heat the coconut oil in large sauté pan on medium-high.

2. Cook the sweet potatoes in the hot oil for 7 minutes, stirring often.

3. Once brown, sprinkle the potatoes with cinnamon and serve.

PER SERVING: Calories: 116 | Fat: 7 g | Protein: 1.5 g | Sodium: 36 mg | Fiber: 2 g | Carbohydrates: 13 g | Sugar: 4 g | GI: Moderate

Sautéed Brussels Sprouts

Brussels sprouts will no longer be boring when they are spiced up with bacon and garlic. These are a great appetizer or side dish for any main meal.

INGREDIENTS | SERVES 4

4 cups fresh Brussels sprouts

2 tablespoons olive oil

½ cup minced shallots

½ cup sliced mushrooms

4 cloves garlic, minced

3 ounces uncured, nitrate-free bacon, diced

1. In a large pot add 1 cup of water and steam Brussels sprouts over medium-high heat until tender, about 10 minutes.

2. Heat the olive oil in a medium frying pan over medium heat. Sauté the shallots, mushrooms, and garlic until caramelized, approximately 5 minutes. Remove from pan.

3. In the same pan, cook the bacon until crisp.

4. Add the Brussels sprouts mixture to the bacon and cook over medium heat for 5 minutes. Remove from heat and serve.

PER SERVING: Calories: 141 | Fat: 7.5 g | Protein: 5 g | Sodium: 37 mg | Fiber: 4 g | Carbohydrates: 19 g | Sugar: 5 g | GI: Moderate

Colcannon

A traditional Irish potato and cabbage recipe, this side dish is an incredibly healthful way to include more vitamin-rich leafy green vegetables in your diet.

INGREDIENTS | SERVES 6

2½ pounds organic russet potatoes (about 4 large), peeled and cut into large chunks

1 teaspoon salt

6 tablespoons butter

3 cups chopped green cabbage (or organic kale, chard, or other leafy green)

1 cup whole milk

3 green onions, sliced

A Frugal Main Dish

Colcannon is often eaten with boiled ham or Irish bacon and is a staple in some Irish homes. The greens used for the dish are normally kale or cabbage, depending on what's available seasonally. Both of these greens are extremely affordable and healthful food sources and can also be stretched in soups and stews. An old Irish holiday tradition was to serve Colcannon with small gold coins hidden in it.

1. Add the potatoes to a medium pot on the stove. Cover with cold water and add salt. Bring to a boil. Cook the potatoes over medium-high heat until they are fork-tender, about 10–15 minutes. Drain the potatoes and add them to a greased 4-quart slow cooker.

2. Add the butter and chopped greens to the slow cooker. Stir them into the potatoes.

3. Cover and cook on low for 4–5 hours or on high for 2½–3 hours.

4. An hour before serving, stir the milk into the potatoes, and mash the potatoes into the greens with a fork. Sprinkle with green onions about 15 minutes before serving.

PER SERVING: Calories: 266 | Fat: 13 g | Protein: 5 g | Sodium: 430.5 mg | Fiber: 5.5 g | Carbohydrates: 33.5 g | Sugar: 6 g | GI: Moderate

CHAPTER 21

Snacks

Chicken Nuggets

These chicken nuggets are fantastic for kids and adults.
Mix them in a green salad or serve with sweet potato fries.

INGREDIENTS | SERVES 4

2 boneless, skinless chicken breasts, cut into bite-size pieces
½ cup olive oil
4 cloves garlic, minced
¼ teaspoon freshly ground black pepper
½ cup almond flour

1. Place chicken in a shallow dish.

2. In a small bowl, mix the olive oil, garlic, and pepper. Pour over the chicken and marinate for 30 minutes in the refrigerator.

3. Preheat the oven to 475°F.

4. Place the almond flour in a shallow bowl. Remove the chicken from the marinade and dredge in almond flour to coat.

5. Bake in a baking dish for 10 minutes or until brown.

PER SERVING: Calories: 369 | Fat: 28 g | Protein: 20 g | Sodium: 2 mg | Fiber: 2 g | Carbohydrates: 12 g | Sugar: 2 g | GI: Very low

Stuffed Mushroom Caps

These appetizers are a bit more exciting than traditional breadcrumb recipes. They are stuffed with protein and fats to ensure more macronutrients in each bite.

INGREDIENTS | SERVES 10

20 button mushrooms
2 tablespoons walnut oil or olive oil
½ pound chopped ground turkey
4 cloves garlic, minced
½ cup finely chopped walnuts
½ teaspoon freshly ground black pepper

1. Preheat the oven to 350°F.

2. Remove stems and hollow out the mushroom caps. Dice the stems and place them in a medium bowl.

3. Heat the walnut oil in a medium frying pan, and cook the ground turkey and garlic for 5–8 minutes, or until the turkey is no longer pink.

4. Add the mushrooms, walnuts, and pepper to the ground turkey, and cook until the mushrooms are soft, about 8 minutes.

5. Stuff the turkey mixture into the mushroom caps and place on a cookie sheet.

6. Bake 20 minutes or until golden brown on top.

PER SERVING: Calories: 88 | Fat: 7 g | Protein: 7 g | Sodium: 2 mg | Fiber: 1 g | Carbohydrates: 2 g | Sugar: 1 g | GI: Very low

Balsamic Almonds

These sweet-and-sour almonds are a great addition to a cheese platter or appetizer plate.

INGREDIENTS | SERVES 15

2 cups whole almonds
½ cup dark brown sugar
½ cup balsamic vinegar
½ teaspoon kosher salt

Healthful Almonds

Botanically speaking, almonds are a seed, not a nut. They are an excellent source of vitamin E and have high levels of monounsaturated fat, one of the two "good" fats responsible for lowering LDL cholesterol.

1. Place all the ingredients into a 4-quart slow cooker. Cook uncovered on high for 4 hours, stirring every 15 minutes or until all the liquid has evaporated. The almonds will have a syrupy coating.

2. Line two cookie sheets with parchment paper. Pour the almonds in a single layer on the baking sheets to cool completely. Store in an airtight container in the pantry for up to 2 weeks.

PER SERVING: Calories: 108 | Fat: 6 g | Protein: 3 g | Sodium: 83 mg | Fiber: 1.5 g | Carbohydrates: 11 g | Sugar: 9 g | GI: Low

Scallops Wrapped in Bacon

This common party appetizer has been revamped with nitrate-free bacon. You are sure to like these much better than the old unhealthy version.

INGREDIENTS | SERVES 10

2 tablespoons olive oil
20 large scallops
2 tablespoons minced garlic
20 slices uncured, nitrate-free bacon

1. Heat the olive oil in a large frying pan over medium-high heat. Sauté the scallops in the oil with the garlic until the scallops are lightly browned. Remove scallops and garlic and set aside to cool.

2. Cook the bacon slightly on each side in the same frying pan and use it to wrap the scallops. Do not overcook the bacon or it will not wrap around the scallops.

3. Secure each appetizer with a toothpick and serve warm.

PER SERVING: Calories: 159 | Fat: 15 g | Protein: 13 g | Sodium: 291 mg | Fiber: 0 g | Carbohydrates: 0 g | Sugar: 0 g | GI: Zero

Roasted Spicy Pumpkin Seeds

*This spicy seed recipe is sure to be a favorite snack for the family.
It is quick to prepare and easy to grab for on-the-go snacks.*

INGREDIENTS | SERVES 6

3 cups raw pumpkin seeds
½ cup olive oil
½ teaspoon garlic powder
Freshly ground black pepper to taste

Pumpkin Seed Benefits

Pumpkin seeds have great health benefits.
They contain L-tryptophan, a compound
found to naturally fight depression, and are
high in zinc, a mineral that protects against
osteoporosis.

1. Preheat the oven to 200°F.

2. In a medium bowl, mix the pumpkin seeds, olive oil, garlic powder, and black pepper until the pumpkin seeds are evenly coated.

3. Spread them in an even layer on a cookie sheet.

4. Bake for 1 hour and 15 minutes, stirring every 10–15 minutes until the seeds are toasted.

PER SERVING: Calories: 532 | Fat: 50 g | Protein: 17 g | Sodium: 13 mg | Fiber: 3 g | Carbohydrates: 12 g | Sugar: 1 g | GI: Very low

Apple Oatmeal Bars

These easy oatmeal bars filled with fresh fruit can also be served as a less-sugary dessert.

INGREDIENTS | SERVES 9

¾ cup brown rice flour

¾ cup arrowroot starch

1 teaspoon baking powder

¼ teaspoon salt

1½ cups gluten-free rolled oats

⅓ cup organic sucanat sugar, packed (found at a natural grocery store)

¾ cup coconut oil or butter

2–3 small organic apples, any variety, seeds removed, coarsely chopped or grated

2 teaspoons ground cinnamon

½ teaspoon ground nutmeg

¼ cup sugar

1 tablespoon honey

Fruit Bar Variations

If you're not a fan of apples, use peaches, pears, blueberries, or other berries in place of the apples. You could also substitute 1 cup of pumpkin purée, butternut squash purée, or even cooked and mashed sweet potatoes.

1. Preheat oven to 350°F. Grease an 8" × 8" baking dish with olive oil, or line with parchment paper.

2. In a large bowl, whisk the brown rice flour, arrowroot starch, baking powder, salt, rolled oats, and organic sucanat sugar. Using a pastry blender or a knife and fork, cut in the coconut oil or butter until it resembles small peas throughout the mixture. Mix with a fork until you have a crumbly dough. Press half of the mixture into the bottom of the baking dish.

3. In a small saucepan, mix the chopped apples, cinnamon, nutmeg, sugar, and honey. Cook on medium heat for 8–10 minutes, stirring every few minutes until the sugar is completely dissolved and the apples are soft. Pour the apple mixture over the dough in the baking dish.

4. Sprinkle the remaining crumbly dough mixture evenly over the apples.

5. Bake for 30–40 minutes until the tops of the bars are golden brown. Allow the bars to cool completely before cutting.

6. Store any remaining bars in an airtight container in the refrigerator for 2–3 days.

PER SERVING: Calories: 356 | Fat: 16 g | Protein: 3 g | Sodium: 125 mg | Fiber: 3 g | Carbohydrates: 50 g | Sugar: 20 g | GI: Low

Carrot Cake Bread

This is a very lightly sweetened, low-glycemic version of carrot cake.
This bread would make a perfect breakfast on weekday mornings.
Just toast it, and spread it lightly with cream cheese or your favorite low-sugar jam.

INGREDIENTS | MAKES 2 (7½" × 3½") LOAVES

2¼ cups blanched almond flour

¾ cup arrowroot starch or tapioca starch

½ teaspoon ground cinnamon

¼ teaspoon sea salt

1¼ teaspoons baking soda

2 tablespoons melted butter or coconut oil

¾ cup coconut palm sugar or organic sucanat sugar

3 large eggs

2 cups shredded carrots

½ cup almond milk or other nondairy milk

½ teaspoon apple cider vinegar

½ cup raisins (optional)

1. Preheat the oven to 350°F. Heavily grease 2 (7½" × 3½") loaf pans with coconut oil or butter.

2. In a medium bowl, whisk the almond flour, arrowroot starch, cinnamon, sea salt, and baking soda. Set aside. In a large bowl, mix the melted butter, coconut sugar, eggs, carrots, almond milk, and apple cider vinegar. Stir the whisked dry ingredients into the wet ingredients. Fold in the raisins, if desired.

3. Divide the batter evenly between the pans. Bake for 35–40 minutes until a toothpick inserted in the middle comes out clean and the tops of the loaves are golden brown.

4. Allow the loaves to cool on a wire rack for 1 hour before slicing and serving. Wrap leftover bread in plastic wrap and store in zippered bags in the freezer for up to 1 month.

PER SERVING ⅛ LOAF): Calories: 186 | Fat: 10 g | Protein: 5 g | Sodium: | Fiber: 2 g | Carbohydrates: 20 g | Sugar: 11 g | GI: Moderate

Rosemary Basil Crackers

*This versatile recipe can make crispy, crunchy crackers or a cracker-like pizza crust.
Either is delicious and incredibly easy to make.*

INGREDIENTS | MAKES 30 SMALL CRACKERS

1¾ cups plus additional blanched almond flour

½ teaspoon sea salt

1 teaspoon dried, crushed rosemary

1 teaspoon dried basil

2 tablespoons olive oil

1 large egg or equivalent egg replacer

Crispy Pizza Crust

To make this recipe into a pizza crust, make the dough as described in the recipe. Roll the dough into an 11" × 11" circle. Prebake the crust at 350°F for 10 minutes until it's just crispy. Add toppings and bake an additional 10–12 minutes until the toppings have heated through. Allow to cool for 5 minutes and then cut and serve with salad. Cut pizza into 6–8 slices. Yields 1 (12") pizza crust.

1. Preheat the oven to 350°F.

2. In a medium mixing bowl, whisk the almond flour, sea salt, rosemary, and basil.

3. Make a well in the center of the dry ingredients and add the olive oil and egg, mixing thoroughly until you have a stiff dough.

4. Place a 12" × 16" sheet of parchment paper on a large baking sheet. Lightly sprinkle almond flour over the parchment paper and place the dough in the middle, on top of the flour. Place a sheet of plastic wrap gently over the dough as a barrier between the dough and the rolling pin. Roll to ¼" thickness or roughly into a 10" × 14" rectangle. Score the crackers by gently rolling a pizza cutter over the dough in a crisscross pattern to create about 30–40 (1") squares.

5. For the crackers, bake for 12–15 minutes until crackers are lightly golden brown around the edges. Remove the pan from the oven and allow the crackers to cool for 20 minutes before breaking them apart. Cool completely on the parchment paper and store any leftover crackers in an airtight container for up to 1 week on the counter. Baked crackers will freeze well for up to 2 months in an airtight container.

PER SERVING (⅙ RECIPE): Calories: 239 | Fat: 21 g | Protein: 8 g | Sodium: 208 mg | Fiber: 3.5 g | Carbohydrates: 7 g | Sugar: 1 g | GI: Very low

Stuffed Celery

This unique take on stuffed celery is wonderful, replacing peanut butter or cream cheese with luxurious, buttery Brie.

INGREDIENTS | SERVES 12

Wide ends of 6 celery stalks, cut in half

5 ounces Brie cheese, softened

2 tablespoons capers

3 tablespoons chopped walnuts, toasted

1. Lay the celery pieces on a cool serving plate. Remove the skin from the Brie and mash with a fork. Mix in the capers.

2. Stuff each piece of celery with the filling and garnish with toasted walnuts.

PER SERVING: Calories: 66 | Fat: 6 g | Protein: 3 g | Sodium: 131 mg | Carbohydrates: 1 g | Sugar: 0.5 g | GI: Low

Wild Rice with Walnuts and Apples

This is a wonderful snack and is very filling. It also makes a great side dish.

INGREDIENTS | SERVES 4

2 cups wild rice, soaked in warm water overnight and cooked to package directions

2 shallots

1 tart organic apple, peeled, cored, and chopped

¼ cup olive oil

½ cup walnuts, toasted

Salt and pepper to taste

While the rice is cooking, sauté the shallots and apple in the olive oil in a medium frying pan on medium heat for 5 minutes. Mix all the ingredients together in a large bowl and serve immediately.

PER SERVING: Calories: 417 | Fat: 32 g | Protein: 8 g | Sodium: 347 mg | Fiber: 4 g | Carbohydrates: 31 g | Sugar: 5 g | GI: Very low

Skewered Chicken Satay with Baby Eggplants

This combination of grilled vegetables, chicken, and Asian flavors is delicious and complemented by the easy-to-make almond dipping sauce.

INGREDIENTS | SERVES 4

12 bamboo skewers, soaked in water for 1 hour

1 pound boneless, skinless chicken breasts, cut into bite-size chunks

2 baby eggplants, cut in half lengthwise, unpeeled

¼ cup lemon juice

½ cup gluten-free soy sauce, divided

Salt and pepper to taste

½ cup almond butter

1 tablespoon pineapple juice

1 teaspoon Tabasco

1 head romaine lettuce leaves (save small white hearts for salad)

1. Skewer the chicken and eggplants on separate skewers. Mix the lemon juice, ¼ cup of soy sauce, salt, and pepper in a bowl. Brush the mixture on the eggplant halves first, and then on the chicken.

2. Set the grill on medium or use the broiler on high.

3. Make the almond dipping sauce by mixing the almond butter, remaining soy sauce, pineapple juice, and Tabasco. If the sauce is too thick, add more pineapple juice.

4. Grill the chicken and eggplants for 4–5 minutes per side, turning frequently.

5. Dip the skewered chicken and eggplant in peanut dipping sauce to serve. Use the lettuce leaves as wraps to prevent burning your hands or getting sticky.

PER SERVING: Calories: 438 | Fat: 24 g | Protein: 51 g | Sodium: 600 mg | Fiber: 2 g | Carbohydrates: 11 g | Sugar: 3 g | GI: Very low

Steak and Mushroom Kebabs

These meaty, juicy kabobs are a hit at summer barbecues.
They can also be cooked indoors on a well-seasoned grilling pan.

INGREDIENTS | SERVES 3

1 pound sirloin steak
3 tablespoons olive oil
¼ cup balsamic vinegar
1 tablespoon Worcestershire sauce
½ teaspoon salt
2 cloves garlic, minced
Freshly ground black pepper to taste
½ pound large white mushrooms

1. Cut the steak into 1½" cubes.

2. Combine the oil, vinegar, Worcestershire sauce, salt, garlic, and pepper to make a marinade.

3. Wash the mushrooms and cut them in half. Place the steak and mushrooms in a shallow bowl with the marinade in the refrigerator for 1–2 hours.

4. Place the mushrooms and steak cubes on separate wooden or metal skewers. Grill at 350°F for about 4 minutes per side for medium-rare steak. You may need additional cooking time for the mushrooms.

PER SERVING: Calories: 321 | Fat: 17 g | Protein: 25 g | Sodium: 401 mg | Fiber: 2 g | Carbohydrates: 16 g | Sugar: 1 g | GI: Low

CHAPTER 22

Desserts

Baked Apples

*You will feel as if you're eating apple pie when you eat these,
and your house will smell like Thanksgiving dinner.*

INGREDIENTS | SERVES 6

6 organic Pink Lady apples
1 cup unsweetened coconut flakes
Ground cinnamon to taste

1. Preheat the oven to 350°F.

2. Remove the cores to within ½" of the bottom of the apples.

3. Place the apples in a medium baking dish.

4. Fill the cores with coconut flakes and sprinkle with cinnamon.

5. Bake for 10–15 minutes. Apples are done when they are completely soft and brown on top.

PER SERVING: Calories: 159 | Fat: 9.5 g | Protein: 1 g | Sodium: 6.5 mg | Fiber: 4.5 g | Carbohydrates: 21 g | Sugar: 5 g | GI: Low

Carrot Nutmeg Pudding

Carrots are often served as a savory side dish. In this recipe,
the carrots have just a little bit of sugar added to bring out their natural sweetness.

INGREDIENTS | SERVES 4

4 large carrots, peeled and grated

2 tablespoons butter

½ teaspoon salt

½ teaspoon freshly grated nutmeg

2 tablespoons sucanat sugar

1 teaspoon vanilla extract

1 cup milk

3 eggs, beaten

1. Add the carrots and butter to a large glass microwavable bowl. Cook on high for 3–4 minutes until the carrots are slightly softened.

2. Stir in the remaining ingredients and pour into a greased 2.5-quart slow cooker. Cook on high for 3 hours or on low for 6 hours. Serve hot or cold.

PER SERVING: Calories: 200 | Fat: 12 g | Protein: 7.5 g | Sodium: 424 mg | Fiber: 2 g | Carbohydrates: 17 g | Sugar: 13.5 g | GI: Moderate

Butternut Squash with Walnuts and Vanilla

Butternut squash has a very mild, slightly sweet flavor. Often people who don't like sweet potatoes enjoy
this as an alternative side dish. Here, it's transformed into a delicious dessert.

INGREDIENTS | SERVES 4

1 butternut squash (about 2 pounds), peeled, seeds removed, and cut into 1" cubes

½ cup water

½ cup organic sucanat sugar (found at a natural grocery store)

1 cup chopped walnuts

1 teaspoon ground cinnamon

4 tablespoons butter

2 teaspoons grated fresh ginger

1 teaspoon vanilla

1. Grease a 4-quart slow cooker with butter. Add the cubed butternut squash and water to the slow cooker.

2. In a small bowl, mix the organic sucanat sugar, walnuts, cinnamon, butter, ginger, and vanilla. Sprinkle this mixture evenly over the squash.

3. Cook on high for 4 hours or on low for 6–8 hours, or until the butternut squash is fork-tender.

PER SERVING: Calories: 468 | Fat: 30 g | Protein: 6 g | Sodium: 16 mg | Fiber: 5 g | Carbohydrates: 48 g | Sugar: 30 g | GI: Moderate

Vanilla-Poached Pears

Slow poaching makes these pears meltingly tender and infuses them with a rich vanilla flavor.

INGREDIENTS | SERVES 4

4 organic Bosc pears, peeled
1 vanilla bean, split
2 tablespoons vanilla extract
2 cups water or organic apple juice

In a Pinch . . .

If you need an easy dessert but don't have fresh fruit, use a large can of sliced or halved pears. Drain and rinse them thoroughly. Make the recipe as written, except use only ½ cup of water or apple juice.

1. Stand the pears up in a 4-quart slow cooker. Add the remaining ingredients.

2. Cook on low for 2 hours or until the pears are tender. Discard all cooking liquid prior to serving.

PER SERVING: Calories: 115 | Fat: 0 g | Protein: 1 g | Sodium: 6 mg | Fiber: 5 g | Carbohydrates: 26 g | Sugar: 17 g | GI: Low

Almond Butter Cookies

Almond cookies are a great snack. They contain the essential fatty acids omega-6 and omega-3. Almonds are also a source of vitamin E.

INGREDIENTS | SERVES 12

1 cup almond butter
1 large egg white
2 tablespoons unsweetened organic applesauce
2 tablespoons unsweetened coconut flakes
1 tablespoon cacao powder

Using the Yolk

If a recipe calls for using just the egg white, as this one does, don't throw out the yolk! You can use it to make mayonnaise. There are important vitamins including choline and B$_{12}$ in the yolk.

1. Preheat the oven to 375°F.

2. Beat all the ingredients together to form a thick batter.

3. Place tablespoon-size scoops of dough onto an ungreased cookie sheet. Bake 10–12 minutes or until lightly brown on top.

PER SERVING: Calories: 151 | Fat: 14 g | Protein: 3.8 g | Sodium: 8.6 mg | Fiber: 1.5 g | Carbohydrates: 5.5 g | Sugar: 3 g | GI: Low

Grain-Free Chocolate Chunk Cookies

Even when you follow a low-glycemic diet, you should allow yourself treats occasionally. These high-protein, low-carb cookies are a great alternative to the sugar-filled and wheat-laden chocolate chip cookies you used to eat. Plus, they are very easy to make!

INGREDIENTS | MAKES 12 COOKIES

2 cups blanched almond flour

½ cup coconut palm sugar or sucanat sugar

3 tablespoons arrowroot starch or tapioca starch

½ teaspoon baking soda

2 heaping tablespoons ground flaxseeds (optional)

¼ teaspoon sea salt

3 tablespoons coconut oil or butter

1 tablespoon vanilla extract

1 teaspoon almond extract

3–4 tablespoons almond milk or water, as needed

1 (3.5-ounce) 70% dark chocolate bar, chopped into chunks

A Few Tips

Do not try to make these cookies with left-over almond pulp from homemade almond milk. It doesn't work—the pulp is too wet and doesn't set up while baking. Instead of coconut palm sugar or sucanat sugar, you can use regular sugar, brown sugar, or honey in these cookies.

1. Preheat the oven to 350°F. Line a large cookie sheet with parchment paper.

2. In a large bowl, whisk the almond flour, coconut palm sugar, arrowroot starch, baking soda, flaxseeds, and salt. Cut the coconut oil or butter into the dry ingredients with a pastry blender or a knife and fork until the shortening resembles very small peas evenly throughout the dry ingredients.

3. Make a well in the center of the dry ingredients and add the vanilla extract, almond extract, and 3 tablespoons of almond milk. Using a little elbow grease, stir the wet ingredients into the dry ingredients until you have a very thick batter (it might be a bit crumbly).

4. This may take several minutes to incorporate well. If necessary, use an additional tablespoon of almond milk, but don't add too much milk or the cookies will not turn out right. Fold in the chopped chocolate chunks and evenly mix them throughout the dough. Scoop the dough into golf ball–size mounds and place on cookie sheet about 2" apart. Flatten lightly and shape with your hands into round cookies.

5. Bake for 12–15 minutes depending on how crispy you want your cookies. The edges should be golden brown when done. Store leftovers in an airtight container on the counter or in the refrigerator for 2–3 days. These cookies are best the day they are made.

PER SERVING (1 COOKIE): Calories: 191 | Fat: 13 g | Protein: 4 g | Sodium: 102 mg | Fiber: 2 g | Carbohydrates: 16 g | Sugar: 11 g | GI: Low

Chocolate–Coconut Milk Balls

These coconut milk balls are not as creamy as ice cream, but they are a nice alternative. You can change the flavor by changing the fruit purée that you add to the recipe.

INGREDIENTS | SERVES 10

12 tablespoons raw cacao powder

6 tablespoons fresh fruit purée of your choice

6 tablespoons coconut oil

6 tablespoons coconut milk

3 tablespoons unsweetened shredded coconut

2 tablespoons cacao nibs

1 ripe banana

1. Combine all the ingredients in a food processor and pulse until very smooth.

2. Add water if the consistency is not fluid.

3. Pour into ice-cube trays or molds and freeze.

PER SERVING: Calories: 149 | Fat: 13 g | Protein: 2 g | Sodium: 4 mg | Fiber: 3.5 g | Carbohydrates: 11 g | Sugar: 6 g | GI: Low

Coconut

Coconut has many great properties. This recipe uses all the edible parts of the coconut—the meat, oil, and milk. Coconut provides high amounts of fiber, vitamins, and minerals as well as being good for your skin.

Grain-Free Chocolate Bars

Your kids will be thrilled when they see these chocolate bars in their lunchboxes. These bars are quick to whip up and quick to eat. The amount of honey can be varied depending on your desired level of sweetness.

INGREDIENTS | SERVES 8

1 tablespoon raw honey
4 tablespoons coconut oil
¼ cup ground almonds
¼ cup ground hazelnuts
¼ cup sunflower seeds
¼ cup cacao powder
¾ cups shredded unsweetened coconut flakes

1. Melt the honey and coconut oil in medium saucepan over medium heat.

2. In a large mixing bowl, combine the almonds, hazelnuts, sunflower seeds, cacao powder, and coconut. Mix thoroughly.

3. Add the honey mixture to the bowl and mix well.

4. Pour the dough into an 8" × 8" baking pan and store in the refrigerator or freezer until firm, about 10 minutes.

5. Cut into squares and enjoy.

PER SERVING (1 SQUARE): Calories: 154 | Fat: 15 g | Protein: 2 g | Sodium: 2 mg | Fiber: 2 g | Carbohydrates: 5 g | Sugar: 4 g | GI: Low

APPENDIX A

References

Chapter 1

Kjellberg, S.R. et al. "The Effect of Adrenaline on the Contraction of the Human Heart under Normal Circulatory Conditions." *Acta Physiologica Scandinavica*, Nov. 1952, 24(4): 333–349.

Whitworth, J.A. et al. "Cardiovascular Consequences of Cortisol Excess." *Vasc. Health Risk Manag.*, Dec. 2005, 1(4): 291–299.

Powell, Dirk. *Endocrinology and Naturopathic Therapies, 8th ed.*, 2008.

Chapter 2

Oosterholt, B.G. "Burnout and Cortisol: Evidence for a Lower Cortisol Awakening Response in Both Clinical and Non-Clinical Burnout." *J. Psychosom. Res.*, Nov. 8, 2014.

Rimer, Sara, and Drexler, Madeline. "Happiness and Health." *Harvard Public Health*, Winter 2011, *www.hsph.harvard.edu/news/magazine/happiness-stress-heart-disease/*.

McGonigal, Kelly. "How to Make Stress Your Friend." TED talk, Sept. 2013, *http://kellymcgonigal.com/*.

Chapter 3

Prasad, R. et al. "Oxidative Stress and Adrenocortical Insufficiency." *J. Endocrinol.*, June 2014, 221(3): R63–R73.

Adly, Amira A.M. "Oxidative Stress and Disease: An Updated Review." *Res. J. Immun.*, Oct. 8, 2010, 3: 129–145.

Pham-Huy, L.H. et al. "Free Radicals, Antioxidants in Disease and Health." *Int. J. Biomed. Sci.,* June 2008, 4(2): 89–96.

Uttara, B. et al. "Oxidative Stress and Neurodegenerative Diseases: A Review of Upstream and Downstream Antioxidant Therapeutic Options." *Curr. Neuropharmacol.,* Mar. 2009, 7(1): 65–74.

Chapter 4

Tops, M. et al. "The Psychobiology of Burnout: Are There Two Different Syndromes?" *Neuropsychobiology,* 2007, 55(3–4): 143–150.

Chapter 5

Kulkarni, S. et al. "Stress and Hypertension." *Wisc. Med. J.,* Dec. 1998, 97(11): 34–38.

Gu, Qiuping et al. "Trends in Antihypertensive Medication Use and Blood Pressure Control Among United States Adults With Hypertension." *Circulation,* 2012, 126: 2105–2114.

The American Institute of Stress. "Stress and Hypertension: Symptoms and Treatment," *www.stress.org/hypertension/.*

Malik, Marek. "Heart Rate Variability." *Circulation,* 1996, 93: 1043–1065.

Anxiety and Depression Association of America. "Tips to Manage Anxiety and Stress," *www.adaa.org/tips-manage-anxiety-and-stress.*

Chetty, S. et al. "Stress and Glucocorticoids Promote Oligodendrogenesis in the Adult Hippocampus." *Molecular Psychiatry,* Dec. 2014, 19: 1275–1283.

Kirby, E.D. et al. "Acute Stress Enhances Adult Rat Hippocampal Neurogenesis and Activation of Newborn Neurons via Secreted Astrocytic FGF2." *eLife*, 2013; 2:e00362, *http://elifesciences.org/content/2/e00362*.

Chapter 7

Budkevich, R.O. et al. "Effects of Nighttime Snacking in Students on Their Physiological Parameters." *Vopr Pitan,* 2014, 83(3): 17–24.

Chapter 9

Jin, P. "Efficacy of Tai Chi, Brisk Walking, Meditation, and Reading in Reducing Mental and Emotional Stress." *J. Psychosom. Res.*, May 1992, 36(4): 361–370.

Jin, P. "Changes in Heart Rate, Noradrenaline, Cortisol and Mood During Tai Chi." *J. Psychosom. Res.*, 1989, 33(2): 197–206.

Pickut, B.A. et al. "Mindfulness Based Intervention in Parkinson's Disease Leads to Structural Brain Changes on MRI: A Randomized Controlled Longitudinal Trial." *Clin. Neurol. Neurosurg.*, Dec. 2013, 115(12): 2419–2425.

Chevalier, G. et al. "Earthing: Health Implications of Reconnecting the Human Body to the Earth's Surface Electrons." *J. Environ. Public Health*, 2012, 2012: 291541.

Tharion, E. et al. "Influence of Deep Breathing Exercise on Spontaneous Respiratory Rate and Heart Rate Variability: A Randomised Controlled Trial in Healthy Subjects." *Indian J. Physiol. Pharmacol.*, Jan.–Mar. 2012, 56(1): 80–87.

Sivakumar, G. et al. "Acute Effects of Deep Breathing for a Short Duration (2–10 Minutes) on Pulmonary Functions in Healthy Young Volunteers." *Indian J. Physiol. Pharmacol.,* Apr.–June 2011, 55(2): 154–159.

Diaz-Rodriguez, L. et al. "Immediate Effects of Reiki on Heart Rate Variability, Cortisol Levels, and Body Temperature in Health Care Professionals with Burnout." *Biol. Res. Nurs.,* Oct. 2011, 13(4): 376–382.

Jain, S. et al. "Healing Touch with Guided Imagery for PTSD in Returning Active Duty Military: A Randomized Controlled Trial." *Mil. Med.,* Sept. 2012, 177(9): 1015–1021.

Chapter 10

Padayatty, S.J. et al. "Human Adrenal Glands Secrete Vitamin C in Response to Adrenocorticotrophic Hormone." *Am. J. Clin. Nutr.,* July 2007, 86(1): 145–149.

Wintergerst, E.S. et al. "Immune-Enhancing Role of Vitamin C and Zinc and Effect on Clinical Conditions." *Ann. Nutr. Metab.,* 2006, 50(2): 85–94.

APPENDIX B

Additional Resources

Books

Conscious Loving: The Journey to Co-Commitment
Gay Hendricks, PhD, and Kathlyn Hendricks, PhD

Nonviolent Communication: A Language of Life
Marshall B. Rosennerg, PhD

The Brain That Changes Itself: Stories of Personal Triumph from the Frontiers of Brain Science
Norman Doidge, MD

Eat Fat Lose Fat: The Healthy Alternative to Trans Fats
Dr. Mary Enig & Sally Fallon

The Total Money Makeover: A Proven Plan for Financial Fitness
Dave Ramsey

Total Wellness: Improve Your Health by Understanding and Cooperating with Your Body's Natural Healing Systems
Joseph Pizzorno, ND

Hormone Deception: How Our Environment (Home, Office, Food, Air and Water) Deceives Our Hormones—and How to Protect Yourself and Your Family
D. Lindsey Berkson

Cookbooks

Nourishing Traditions: The Cookbook That Challenges Politically Correct Nutrition and the Diet Dictocrats
Sally Fallon

Gut and Psychology Syndrome: Natural Treatment for Autism, Dyspraxia, A.D.D., Dyslexia, A.D.H.D., Depression, Schizophrenia
Dr. Natasha Campbell-McBride, MD

Keto Clarity: Your Definitive Guide to the Benefits of a Low-Carb, High-Fat Diet
Jimmy Moore with Eric C. Westman, MD

Healing with Whole Foods: Asian Traditions and Modern Nutrition
Paul Pitchford

The Art of Fermentation: An In-Depth Exploration of Essential Concepts and Processes from around the World
Sandor Ellix Katz

Places to Buy Bulk Herbs Online

Mountain Rose
www.mountainroseherbs.com

Starwest Botanicals
www.starwest-botanicals.com

Websites

www.stress.org
www.diagnostechs.com/Pages/AdrenalStressIndex.aspx
www.greatplainslaboratory.com/home/eng/hormones.asp
http://biohealthlab.com/test-menu/hormones/functional-adrenal-stress-profiles/
www.23andme.com
www.holisticheal.com/dna-methylation-pathway-test-kit.html
http://yourwellnessexpert.com
www.nongmoproject.org
www.organicconsumers.org/taxonomy/term/235/0
www.localharvest.org/csa/
www.ewg.org

Trusted Supplement Companies

www.seekinghealth.com
www.newchapter.com
www.designsforhealth.com
www.xymogen.com
www.integrativepro.com
www.metabolicmaintenance.com
www.herb-pharm.com
www.gaiaherbs.com
https://thorne.com
www.douglaslabs.com
www.pureencapsulations.com
www.vitalnutrients.net
www.allergyresearchgroup.com

Standard U.S./Metric Measurement Conversions

VOLUME CONVERSIONS

U.S. Volume Measure	Metric Equivalent
⅛ teaspoon	0.5 milliliter
¼ teaspoon	1 milliliter
½ teaspoon	2 milliliters
1 teaspoon	5 milliliters
½ tablespoon	7 milliliters
1 tablespoon (3 teaspoons)	15 milliliters
2 tablespoons (1 fluid ounce)	30 milliliters
¼ cup (4 tablespoons)	60 milliliters
⅓ cup	90 milliliters
½ cup (4 fluid ounces)	125 milliliters
⅔ cup	160 milliliters
¾ cup (6 fluid ounces)	180 milliliters
1 cup (16 tablespoons)	250 milliliters
1 pint (2 cups)	500 milliliters
1 quart (4 cups)	1 liter (about)

WEIGHT CONVERSIONS

U.S. Weight Measure	Metric Equivalent
½ ounce	15 grams
1 ounce	30 grams
2 ounces	60 grams
3 ounces	85 grams
¼ pound (4 ounces)	115 grams
½ pound (8 ounces)	225 grams
¾ pound (12 ounces)	340 grams
1 pound (16 ounces)	454 grams

OVEN TEMPERATURE CONVERSIONS

Degrees Fahrenheit	Degrees Celsius
200 degrees F	95 degrees C
250 degrees F	120 degrees C
275 degrees F	135 degrees C
300 degrees F	150 degrees C
325 degrees F	160 degrees C
350 degrees F	180 degrees C
375 degrees F	190 degrees C
400 degrees F	205 degrees C
425 degrees F	220 degrees C
450 degrees F	230 degrees C

BAKING PAN SIZES

American	Metric
8 x 1½ inch round baking pan	20 x 4 cm cake tin
9 x 1½ inch round baking pan	23 x 3.5 cm cake tin
11 x 7 x 1½ inch baking pan	28 x 18 x 4 cm baking tin
13 x 9 x 2 inch baking pan	30 x 20 x 5 cm baking tin
2 quart rectangular baking dish	30 x 20 x 3 cm baking tin
15 x 10 x 2 inch baking pan	30 x 25 x 2 cm baking tin (Swiss roll tin)
9 inch pie plate	22 x 4 or 23 x 4 cm pie plate
7 or 8 inch springform pan	18 or 20 cm springform or loose bottom cake tin
9 x 5 x 3 inch loaf pan	23 x 13 x 7 cm or 2 lb narrow loaf or pate tin
1½ quart casserole	1.5 liter casserole
2 quart casserole	2 liter casserole

Index

Note: Page numbers in **bold** indicate recipe category lists.